W9-DGJ-138

Emergency Diagnostic Tests for Cardiac Ischemia

Emergency Diagnostic Tests for Cardiac Ischemia

A Report from
the National Heart Attack Alert Program (NHAAP)
Coordinating Committee:
Working Group on Evaluation of Technologies
for Identifying Acute Cardiac Ischemia
in the Emergency Department

Co-chairs

Harry P. Selker, MD
Chief, Division of Clinical Care Research
Director, Center for Cardiovascular Health Services Research
New England Medical Center
Associate Professor of Medicine
Tufts University School of Medicine
Boston, Massachusetts

Robert J. Zalenski, MD
Associate Professor
Emergency Medicine and Cardiology
Wayne State University School of Medicine
Detroit, Michigan

b

**Blackwell
Science**

Blackwell Science

Editorial offices:

350 Main Street, Malden, Massachusetts 02148, USA

Osney Mead, Oxford OX2 0E1, England

25 John Street, London WC1N 2BL, England

23 Ainslie Place, Edinburgh EH3 6AJ, Scotland

54 University Street, Carlton, Victoria 3053, Australia

Other Editorial Offices:

Arnette Blackwell SA, 224, Boulevard Saint Germain, 75007 Paris, France

Blackwell Wissenschafts-Verlag GmbH Kurfürstendamm 57, 10707 Berlin, Germany

Zehetnergasse 6, A-1140 Vienna, Austria

Distributors:

USA

Blackwell Science, Inc.

Commerce Place

350 Main Street

Malden, Massachusetts 02148

(Telephone orders: 800-215-1000 or
617-388-8250; Fax orders: 617-388-8270)

Canada

Copp Clark Professional

200 Adelaide Street, West, 3rd Floor

Toronto, Ontario M5H 1W7

(Telephone orders: 416-597-1616
1-800-815-9417

fax: 416-597-1617

Australia

Blackwell Science Pty., Ltd.

54 University Street

Carlton, Victoria 3053

(Telephone orders: 03-9347-0300;
fax orders: 03-9349 3016)

Outside North America and Australia

Blackwell Science, Ltd.

c/o Marston Book Services, Ltd.

P.O. Box 269

Abingdon

Oxon OX14 4YN

England

(Telephone orders: 44-01235-465500;
fax orders 44-01235-465555)

Acquisitions: Jim Krosschell

Production: Kevin Sullivan

Manufacturing: Lisa Flanagan

Typeset by Best-set Typesetter Ltd., Hong Kong

Printed and bound by Capital City Press

© 1997 by Blackwell Science, Inc.

Printed in the United States of America

97 98 99 00 5 4 3 2 1

All rights reserved. No part of this book may be reproduced in any form or by any electronic or mechanical means, including information storage and retrieval systems, without permission in writing from the publisher, except by a reviewer who may quote brief passages in a review.

The Blackwell Science logo is a trade mark of Blackwell Science Ltd., registered at the United Kingdom Trade Marks Registry

Library of Congress Cataloging-in-Publication Data

Selker, Harry.

    Emergency diagnostic tests for cardiac ischemia: a report from NIH's National Heart Attack Alert Program / Harry Selker, Robert J. Zalenski.

        p.   cm.

    Includes bibliographical references and index.

    ISBN 0-632-04304-0

    1. Cardiovascular emergencies—Diagnosis.

    2. Myocardial infarction—Diagnosis.

    3. Coronary heart disease—Diagnosis.

    I. Zalenski, Robert J.   II. National Heart Attack Alert Program (U.S.)   III. Title.

    [DNLM: 1. Heart Function Tests.

    2. Myocardial Infarction—diagnosis.

    3. Myocardial Ischemia—diagnosis.

    4. Emergency Medical Services—United States.   5. Evaluation Studies.

    WG 141.5.F9 S466e 1997]

    RC675.S45 1997

    616.1'23025—dc21

    DNLM/DLC

    for Library of Congress   96-52002
                                                  CIP

Contents

Members of the Working Group on the Evaluation of Technologies for Identifying Acute Cardiac Ischemia in the Emergency Department

Harry P. Selker, MD, MSPH
(Co-chair)
Chief, Division of Clinical Care
  Research
Director, Center for
  Cardiovascular Health Services
  Research
New England Medical Center
Associate Professor of Medicine
Tufts University School of
  Medicine
Boston, Massachusetts

Robert J. Zalenski, MD, MA
(Co-chair)
Associate Professor
Emergency Medicine and
  Cardiology
Wayne State University School
  of Medicine
Detroit, Michigan
(formerly of:
Department of Emergency
  Medicine
Cook County Hospital
Chicago, Illinois)

Elliott M. Antman, MD
Director, Samuel A. Levine
  Cardiac Unit
Cardiovascular Division
Brigham and Women's Hospital
Associate Professor of Medicine
Harvard Medical School
Boston, Massachusetts

Tom P. Aufderheide, MD
Associate Professor of Emergency
  Medicine
Department of Emergency
  Medicine
Medical College of Wisconsin
Milwaukee, Wisconsin

Sheilah A. Bernard, MD
Director, Coronary Care
  Unit
Boston City Hospital
Assistant Professor of
  Medicine
Boston University School of
  Medicine
Boston, Massachusetts

MEMBERS OF THE WORKING GROUP

Robert O. Bonow, MD,
Chief, Division of Cardiology
Goldberg Professor of
   Medicine
Northwestern University Medical
   School
Chicago, Illinois

W. Brian Gibler, MD
Director, Center for Emergency
   Care
Department of Emergency
   Medicine
University of Cincinnati Medical
   Center
Richard C. Levy Professor of
   Emergency Medicine and
   Chairman
Department of Emergency
   Medicine
University of Cincinnati College
   of Medicine
Cincinnati, Ohio

Michael D. Hagen, MD
Vice Chairman, Department of
   Family Practice
University of Kentucky Chandler
   Medical Center
Nicholas J. Pisaciano Professor of
   Family Practice
Associate Chair of Academic
   Affairs
University of Kentucky College
   of Medicine
Lexington, Kentucky

Paula Johnson, MD, MPH
Co-Medical Director
Department of Quality
   Management Services
Brigham and Women's
   Hospital

Instructor in Medicine
Harvard Medical School
Boston, Massachusetts

Joseph Lau, MD
Director, Center for Clinical
   Evidence Synthesis
Division of Clinical Care
   Research
New England Medical Center
Associate Professor of Medicine
Tufts University School of
   Medicine
Boston, Massachusetts

Robert A. McNutt, MD
Chairman, Department of
   Medicine
Milwaukee Clinical Campus
Professor of Medicine
University of Wisconsin Medical
   School
Milwaukee, Wisconsin

Joseph Ornato, MD
Professor of Medicine and
   Cardiology
Medical College of Virginia
Richmond, Virginia

J. Sanford Schwartz, MD
Robert D. Eilers Professor of
   Medicine and Health Care
   Management and Economics
School of Medicine
University of Pennsylvania and
   the Warton School
Executive Director, Leonard
   Davis Institute of Health
   Economics
Philadelphia, Pennsylvania

Jane D. Scott, ScD, MSN
Health Services Researcher
National Study Center for
    Trauma and EMS
University of Maryland at
    Baltimore
Baltimore, Maryland
Formerly with the Agency for
    Health Care Policy and
    Research
Rockville, Maryland

Paul A. Tunick, MD
Associate Professor of Clinical
    Medicine
New York University School of
    Medicine
New York, New York

W. Douglas Weaver, MD
Director, Cardiovascular Critical
    Care
University of Washington
    Medical Center
Professor of Medicine
University of Washington
Seattle, Washington

NHLBI Staff

Mary M. Hand, MSPH, RN
Coordinator, National Heart
    Attack Alert Program
Office of Prevention, Education,
    and Control
National Heart, Lung, and Blood
    Institute
National Institutes of Health
Bethesda, Maryland

Michael Horan, MD, ScM
Director, Division of Heart and
    Vascular Diseases
National Heart, Lung, and Blood
    Institute
National Institutes of Health
Bethesda, Maryland

Contract Staff

John Clinton Bradley, MS
ROW Sciences, Inc.
Rockville, Maryland

Pamela A. Christian, RN, MPA
ROW Sciences, Inc.
Rockville, Maryland

National Heart Attack Alert Program Coordinating Committee Member Organizations

Agency for Health Care Policy and Research
American Academy of Family Physicians
American Academy of Insurance Medicine
American Association for Clinical Chemistry, Inc.
American Association of Critical Care Nurses
American Association of Occupational Health Nurses
American College of Cardiology
American College of Chest Physicians
American College of Emergency Physicians
American College of Occupational and Environmental Medicine
American College of Physicians
American College of Preventive Medicine
American Heart Association
American Hospital Association
American Medical Association
American Nurses' Association, Inc.
American Pharmaceutical Association
American Public Health Association
American Red Cross
Association of Black Cardiologists
Centers for Disease Control and Prevention
Department of Defense, Health Affairs
Department of Veterans Affairs
Emergency Nurses Association
Federal Emergency Management Agency
Food and Drug Administration
Health Care Financing Administration
Health Resources and Services Administration

International Association of Emergency Medical Technicians
National Association of Emergency Medical Technicians
National Association of EMS Physicians
National Association of State Emergency Medical Services Directors
National Black Nurses' Association, Inc.
National Center for Health Statistics
National Heart, Lung, and Blood Institute
National Highway Traffic Safety Administration
National Medical Association
NHLBI Ad Hoc Committee on Minority Populations
Society for Academic Emergency Medicine
Society of General Internal Medicine

Acronyms and Terms

ACI	acute cardiac ischemia
ACI-TIPI	acute cardiac ischemia time-insensitive predictive instrument
AMI	acute myocardial infarction
Accuracy	(true positive patients and true negative patients)/all patients
BEPS	Belgian Eminase Prehospital Study
CABG	coronary artery bypass graft
CAD	coronary artery disease
CCU	coronary care unit
CI	confidence interval
CK	creatine kinase
CK-BB	creatine kinase isoenzyme—brain subunit
CK-MB	creatine kinase isoenzyme—cardiac muscle subunit
CK-MM	creatine kinase isoenzyme—skeletal muscle subunit
CMLC	cardiac myosin light chains
cTnI	cardiac troponin-I
cTnT	cardiac troponin-T
DSP	predictive decision support system
ECG	electrocardiogram
ED	emergency department
EMCREG	Emergency Medicine Cardiac Research Group

EMS   emergency medical services

GISSI   Gruppo Italiano per lo Studio Della
           Streptochinasi nell 'Infarto Miocardico

ID3   induced decision tree method; a recursive
           partitioning method

LAD   left anterior descending
LVH   left ventricular hypertrophy

MCPS   Multicenter Chest Pain Study
MITI   myocardial infarction triage and intervention
MRI   magnetic resonance imaging

NHAAP   National Heart Attack Alert Program
NHLBI   National Heart, Lung, and Blood Institute
NIH   National Institutes of Health
Negative   true negatives/all test negatives
 predictive value
^{99m}Tc sestamibi   technetium-99m-sestamibi

Positive   true positives/all test positives
 predictive value

RCA   right coronary artery
ROC curve   receiver-operating characteristic curve: a
           graphic display of the performance of a
           diagnostic test obtained by plotting 100-
           specificity (x axis) against sensitivity
           (y axis) for each possible value of the test
RVI   right ventricular infarction

Sensitivity   portion of patients with proven disease who
           have a positive test; *true positives/(true*
           positives and false negatives)
Specificity   proportion of patients without the disease
           who have a negative test; *true negatives/*
           (true negatives and false positives)
SPECT   single-photon emission computed
           tomography

TIPI	time-insensitive predictive instrument
UAP	unstable angina pectoris
WHO	World Health Organization

Foreword

In creating the National Heart Attack Alert Program (NHAAP) six years ago, the National Heart, Lung, and Blood Institute initiated a national effort to educate health care professionals, patients, and the public about the importance of rapid identification and treatment of patients with symptoms and signs of an acute myocardial infarction. This was in response to developments in treatment of patients with heart attacks, the current standard of which is early reperfusion of the jeopardized muscle through thrombolytic therapy or percutaneous transluminal coronary angioplasty (PTCA), along with other measures to prevent myocardial damage. The clinical trials of thrombolytic therapy (many of which were first done in the 1980s) showed that dramatic reductions in morbidity and mortality were related to the interval between onset of pain and the start of drug therapy.

The NHAAP directed many of its initial efforts to educating emergency department professionals about reviewing and, as necessary, expediting the process of care for suspected heart attack patients once they arrive at the emergency department. The program's initial thrust of improving time to treatment in the emergency department was in response to reported median delays of 70 to 90 minutes in initiating treatment with thrombolytic therapy in this setting. Such delays were and still are a concern, because plans for phased-in public education activities are dependent on expeditious responses by emergency department providers when these patients arrive at the hospital, given that out-of-hospital delays by patients and others in the community already are major barriers to timely treatment. The NHAAP highlighted the importance of analyzing the process of care for patients presenting to emergency

department professionals with symptoms and signs of acute myocardial infarction in its first publication, compiled by the 60 Minutes
to Treatment Working Group (1).

The next important step for improving emergency department
management of these patients is to evaluate the technologies that
assist in achieving early and accurate diagnosis with demonstrated
benefits in outcome. Accordingly, the Working Group on Evaluation of Technologies for Identifying Acute Cardiac Ischemia in the
Emergency Department was formed by the NHAAP's Science Base
Subcommittee to review new and existing diagnostic methods and
technologies that facilitate the early identification of not only
patients with acute myocardial infarction, but more broadly patients
who present with symptoms and signs of acute cardiac ischemia.
This larger group includes patients with unstable angina pectoris
as well as those with acute myocardial infarction, and is thus more
representative of the approximately six million patients with chest
pain or related symptoms who present to emergency departments
annually.

The Working Group's report comprehensively reviews the
quality of the scientific literature concerning 17 technologies for
identifying patients with acute cardiac ischemia in the emergency
department, and evaluates data for each technology that demonstrate its accuracy and effectiveness in actual use. (It should be noted
that methods primarily directed at prognostic or risk stratification
of patients are not included.) The table titled Summary Working
Group Ratings of Diagnostic Technologies for ACI for ED Use (see
Table 1, p. xxiv, or Table 16-1, p. 174) provides an important
overview of the report's scope and conclusions.

With this thorough review, the NHAAP is very pleased to lay
the foundation for our understanding of the up-to-date scientific
evidence supporting the use of these technologies, and to document the need for more research related to the diagnostic performance and especially the clinical impact of these technologies for
the emergency evaluation of patients with chest pain (the second
most frequent reason for visits to emergency departments in 1995
(2)).

The report further helps to shape a key role for the NHAAP—
that of facilitating the development, dissemination, and incorporation into practice of new technologies. As the NHAAP (and others)
undertakes public education efforts nationally, the rapid and accurate identification of patients through the use of these technologies
will serve to better differentiate between those who do and those

who do not require hospitalization—an outcome that is of keen interest in today's health care environment.

Claude Lenfant, MD
Director, National Heart, Lung, and Blood Institute
National Institutes of Health
Chairman, National Heart Attack Alert Program
    Coordinating Committee
Bethesda, Maryland

REFERENCES

1. National Heart Attack Alert Program Coordinating Committee, 60 Minutes to Treatment Working Group. Emergency department: rapid identification and treatment of patients with acute myocardial infarction. *Ann Emerg Med* 1994;23:311–329.
2. Stussman BJ. National Hospital Ambulatory Medical Care Survey: 1995 emergency department summary. Advance data from vital and health statistics; no. 285. Hyattsville, Maryland: National Center for Health Statistics, 1997.

Notice. The indications and dosages of all drugs in this book have been recommended in the medical literature and conform to the practices of the general medical community. The medications described do not necessarily have specific approval by the Food and Drug Administration for use in the diseases and dosages for which they are recommended. The package insert for each drug should be consulted for use and dosage as approved by the FDA. Because standards of usage change, it is advisable to keep abreast of revised recommendations, particularly those concerning new drugs.

Executive Summary

INTRODUCTION AND METHODS

As the most common cause of death in this country, acute myocardial infarction (AMI) has deservedly been the subject of substantial efforts of clinicians, scientists, government and other agencies, and the public in efforts to reduce its devastating impact. Although very significant progress continues to be made, the National Heart, Lung, and Blood Institute (NHLBI) of the National Institutes of Health (NIH) recognized the need for a concerted and coordinated effort to reduce mortality and morbidity in this country from AMI and in 1991 initiated the National Heart Attack Alert Program (NHAAP). This ongoing effort, bringing together scientists, clinicians, and NHLBI staff, with the active participation and leadership of a coordinating committee that includes representatives of 40 professional organizations, has commissioned a number of working groups to review and make recommendations for physicians and other health care providers about issues related to the rapid recognition and response to patients with symptoms and signs of AMI. Recognizing the central and growing role of diagnostic technologies for AMI and for acute cardiac ischemia (ACI) in general (including both unstable angina pectoris [UAP] and AMI) in emergency settings, which represent patients' entry points into the health care system, in 1994 the NHAAP Working Group on Evaluation of Technologies for Identifying Acute Cardiac Ischemia in the Emergency Department was formed to assess the utility of diagnostic technologies for ACI/AMI in the ED. This report summarizes the Working Group's assessment of the diagnostic performance and impact on care of those technologies. The charge by the NHAAP to the Working Group was to use ACI, rather than

AMI, as the diagnostic outcome of interest in the ED. This reflects the fact that identifying only AMI would miss a large number of ED patients at significant and immediate cardiac risk.

The technologies reviewed address the diagnosis of ACI (ie, both AMI and UAP) because this is the condition that must be identified in the treatment of patients with AMI and potential AMI. The review included all such technologies directed at the *diagnosis* of ACI in the ED; methods primarily directed at prognostic or risk stratification of such patients were not included. In this context, to aid the medical community in the use and further evaluation of diagnostic technologies for ACI, this report by the Working Group: 1) comprehensively reviews the important technologies for identifying ACI in the ED setting available at the time of this writing and 2) describes the extent to which there are data for each technology that demonstrate its accuracy and effectiveness in actual use in the ED setting. The Working Group was selected to provide expertise in the areas of cardiology, emergency medicine, general internal medicine, family practice, and nursing, as well as in the specific disciplines of metaanalysis and health services research.

WORKING GROUP PROCESS AND METHODS

To accomplish this review, a formal process of review and evaluation of the scientific literature related to these technologies was undertaken, based on Medline and related electronic literature searches and supplemented by the panelists' knowledge of the literature and ongoing research. All relevant English-language literature on each technology was reviewed, summarized, analyzed, and reported on independently by three panel members in a process analogous to an NIH Study Section.

For each technology, studies were formally evaluated and then rated. The *quality of evidence* provided by the relevant studies was rated as A, B, C, or NK, as follows: A, prospective controlled clinical studies of high quality (eg, large multicenter trials with concurrent controls); B, substantial clinical studies; C, limited studies or evidence (eg, case studies, small clinical studies); and NK, not known (eg, expert opinion or case reports only).

On the basis of compiled initial reviews and a consensus process, the panel rated each technology (in addition to the quality ratings described above) for its primary purpose using two distinct metrics: 1) *diagnostic performance*, the accuracy of the technology, measured by sensitivity, specificity, or receiver-operating characteristic curve, for ACI; and 2) *clinical impact*, its demonstrated impact on diagnosis, triage, treatment, or outcome (eg, mortality) when used by clinicians in actual practice.

The *diagnostic performance* of the test and the magnitude of its demonstrated *clinical impact* were rated as +++, very accurate/large clinical impact; ++, moderately accurate/medium impact; +, modestly accurate/small impact; NK, not known; NE, not effective.

As indicated, in assigning these ratings, each technology was evaluated on the basis of its performance of its *primary* diagnostic purpose of general ED detection (G) early detection (E), and detection in specific subgroup (S). (These designations are noted in Table 1.)

The Working Group's conclusions and ratings for each reviewed diagnostic technology follow. The ratings of the Working Group reflect its estimation of the accuracy or impact of the test in actual practice in the ED. These assessments incorporate the quality of the literature, the magnitude or effect of size of the reported findings, and considerations of generalizability and feasibility. These ratings take into consideration the text of the reviews but also include a weighting of the evidence by the Working Group. Therefore the text and the ratings, although linked, are sometimes not entirely concordant. Full reviews and evaluations of each technology appear in the main body of this report. The key for interpreting the ratings tables is as follows. The quality-of-evidence rating system comprises A, high-quality clinical studies; B, substantial clinical studies; C, limited studies; NK, not known; and NE, not effective. The diagnostic performance and Clinical impact rating system comprises +++, very accurate/large clinical impact; ++, moderately accurate/medium impact; +, modestly accurate/small impact; NK, not known; and NE, not effective.

STANDARD ECG

The ECG represents a safe, readily available, and inexpensive technology for assessing patients with acute chest pain and is central to its evaluation. However, the ECG suffers from imperfect sensitivity and specificity for ACI. When interpreted using liberal criteria, the ECG operates with relatively high (but not perfect) sensitivity for AMI, at the cost of low specificity. Conversely, when interpreted using stringent criteria for AMI, sensitivity drops to levels around 50% or below.

Table 1 Summary Working Group Ratings of Diagnostic Technologies for ACI for ED Use

Technology	Primary Diagnostic Use	ED Diagnostic Performance		Demonstrated ED Clinical Impact	
		Quality of Evidence	Accuracy	Quality of Evidence	Impact
Standard ECG	G	A	++	Standard of care	Standard of care
Original ACI predictive instrument	G	A	+++	A	+++
ACI-TIPI	G	A	+++	C*	+*
Prehospital ECG	E	A	++	B	+
Goldman chest pain protocol	G	A	For AMI: +++ / For UAP: NE	B	NK/NE
CK, multiple tests over time	S	A	For AMI: +++ / For UAP: NE	NK	NK
Sestamibi	S	C	+++	NK	NK
CK, single test	S	A	For AMI: + / For UAP: NE	NK	NK

ECG exercise stress test	S	C	+	C	NK/NE
Echocardiogram	S	B	+	NK	Nk
Other computer-based decision aids	G	B	+	NK	NK
Troponin-T and troponin-I	S	B	For AMI: ++ For UAP: NE	NK	NK
Myoglobin	S	B	For AMI: + For UAP: NE	NK	NK
Nonstandard ECG leads	S	C	+	NK	NK
Thallium scanning	S	C	NK/NE	NK	NK/NE
Body-surface mapping	S	NK	NK	NK	NK
Continuous 12-lead ECG	S	NK	NK	NK	NK

AMI = acute myocardial infarction; **UAP** = unstable angina pectoris; **G** = general detection of ACI; **E** = early detection of ACI; **S** = detection in subgroup. Diagnostic rating: **A** = high-quality clinical studies; **B** = substantial clinical studies; **C** = limited studies; **NK** = not known; **NE** = not effective. Clinical impact rating: +++ = very accurate/large clinical impact; ++ = moderately accurate/medium impact; + = modestly accurate/small impact; **NK** = not known; **NE** = not effective; ★abstract and pending reports are not included in the ratings. Technologies are listed in order of the Working Group's ratings of diagnostic accuracy and demonstrated clinical impact, and alphabetically among equivalent ratings, with the exception of standard ECG, which is considered to be a standard of care.

Table 2 Working Group Ratings of Standard ECG

ED Diagnostic Performance		ED Clinical Impact	
Quality of Evidence	Accuracy	Quality of Evidence	Impact
A	+ +	Standard of care	Standard of care

The ECG depends on a trained interpreter; less experienced ED interpreters appear to operate at lower positive predictive values than trained interpreters. Additionally, the interpreter frequently cannot tell whether ischemic electrocardiographic changes are new or old because previous tracings are not available or changes such as bundle-branch blocks obscure possible new changes. The ECG's yield is greater during active chest pain, and sensitivity may increase.

In spite of these shortcomings, the standard ECG functions as an integral component of the evaluation of patients with acute chest pain and should continue to be incorporated in strategies that incorporate other clinical characteristics such as historical and physical examination parameters. The ECG is not a perfectly sensitive test, and it should always be considered a supplement to, rather than a substitute for, physician judgment. The Working Group recommends the ECG continue to be considered the standard of care in the evaluation of chest pain in the ED patient.

The results of the Working Group's final ratings of the quality of evidence evaluating this technology and of its ED diagnostic performance and clinical impact are depicted in Table 2.

PREHOSPITAL ECG

Studies to date demonstrate that prehospital 12-lead ECG technology is feasible and clinically practical and probably could be implemented in most established urban paramedic systems. *Prehospital identification* of thrombolysis candidates through the use of prehospital 12-lead electrocardiography has been shown in almost every study to significantly reduce hospital-based time to treatment. This time savings is perceived as beneficial but has not, by itself, demonstrated a reduction in mortality. *Prehospital treatment* with thrombolytic therapy may result in a significant mortality reduction if the time savings is in the area of 1 hour or more. Parallel controlled randomized prospective studies are required to further

Table 3 Working Group Ratings Prehospital ECG

ED Diagnostic Performance		ED Clinical Impact	
Quality of Evidence	Accuracy	Quality of Evidence	Impact
A	++	B	+

Table 4 Working Group Ratings of Continuous 12-Lead ECG

ED Diagnostic Performance		ED Clinical Impact	
Quality of Evidence	Accuracy	Quality of Evidence	Impact
NK	NK	NK	NK

analyze the cost-benefit issues, additional uses, and ultimate role of prehospital 12-lead electrocardiography.

The results of the Working Group's final ratings of the quality of evidence evaluating this technology and of its ED diagnostic performance and clinical impact are detailed in Table 3.

CONTINUOUS 12-LEAD ECG

There have been no well-designed large randomized prospective ED or CCU studies evaluating this technology. Cost-benefit analysis of this technology has not been accomplished. Although ED ST-segment monitoring holds the potential to detect silent myocardial ischemia and infarction, reduce missed ischemic diagnoses, and provide the earliest evidence for coronary occlusion in patients presenting with preinfarction angina, larger prospective studies are required to make this assessment.

The results of the Working Group's final ratings of the quality of evidence evaluating this technology and of its ED diagnostic performance and clinical impact are shown in Table 4.

NONSTANDARD ECG LEADS AND
BODY-SURFACE MAPPING

Sampling right ventricular leads is clinically practical, uses the universally available 12-lead ECG, and appears to increase the sensitivity and specificity for detection of right ventricular infarction (a strong, independent predictor of major complications and in-hospital mortality in patients with inferior AMI). Such leads have

Table 5 Working Group Ratings of Nonstandard ECG Leads and Body-Surface Mapping

	ED Diagnostic Performance		ED Clinical Impact	
	Quality of Evidence	Accuracy	Quality of Evidence	Impact
Nonstandard ECG leads	C	+	NK	NK
Body-surface mapping	NK	NK	NK	NK

the potential to improve severity classification of AMIs, help refine the process of risk-benefit assessment for emergency interventions, possibly provide an indication for thrombolytic treatment, and avoid nitrate-induced hypotension in patients with right ventricular infarction. Sampling posterior leads may also improve the sensitivity of the ECG for posterior AMI. Larger prospective studies applied in a variety of EDs with a broader range of admitted and discharged chest pain patients are required to determine the risks and benefits of this technology. If sensitivity and specificity are comparable to the standard 12-lead ECG, then studies to assess clinical impact in the ED would be warranted.

Body-surface mapping is a valuable research tool requiring specialized equipment for acquisition and specialized software for processing the information. This is not currently practical for ED patient assessment. However, the improved sensitivity and specificity suggested by preliminary efficacy-type trials indicate that this approach may eventually contribute to the ED diagnosis of ACI.

The results of the Working Group's final ratings of the quality of evidence evaluating these technologies and of their ED diagnostic performance and clinical impact are detailed in Table 5.

ECG EXERCISE STRESS TEST

Currently there are limited data on the impact of ECG exercise stress testing in the ED. Where the risk of coronary artery disease is low to moderate, the expedited ECG stress test may offer the benefit of an expedited workup and may reduce hospital admissions for chest pain. Observation status, where the patient is observed pending definitive testing, may offer a similar benefit.

Table 6   Working Group Ratings of ECG Exercise Stress Test

ED Diagnostic Performance		ED Clinical Impact	
Quality of Evidence	Accuracy	Quality of Evidence	Impact
C	+	C	NK-NE

However, ECG exercise stress testing in the ED cannot be recommended in the absence of additional data demonstrating safety and effectiveness.

The results of the Working Group's final ratings of the quality of evidence evaluating this technology and of its ED diagnostic performance and clinical impact are shown in Table 6.

ORIGINAL ACI PREDICTIVE INSTRUMENT

The original ACI predictive instrument uses readily available clinical and ECG data to compute a probability of ACI. Its diagnostic performance and clinical impact have been well demonstrated in large prospective clinical trials (1,2), which have shown it to be safe and effective in improving ED triage of patients with possible ACI in a wide range of hospitals. Although appropriate for general clinical use, it has not been widely adopted in EDs, possibly because of the need for a hand-held calculator to compute the probability of ACI.

In the near future, the original ACI predictive instrument probably will be superseded by the ACI-TIPI (time-insensitive predictive instrument), which may have a similar impact on ED care, with the advantages of computerization and its applicability to retrospective review of care.

The results of the Working Group's final ratings of the quality of evidence evaluating this technology and of its ED diagnostic performance and clinical impact are shown in Table 7.

Table 7   Working Group Ratings of Original ACI Predictive Instrument

ED Diagnostic Performance		ED Clinical Impact	
Quality of Evidence	Accuracy	Quality of Evidence	Impact
A	+++	A	+++

Table 8   Working Group Ratings of ACI-TIPI

ED Diagnostic Performance		ED Clinical Impact	
Quality of Evidence	Accuracy	Quality of Evidence	Impact
A	+++	C*	+*

* Abstract and pending reports are not included in the ratings.

ACUTE CARDIAC ISCHEMIA TIME INSENSITIVE PREDICTIVE INSTRUMENT (ACI-TIPI)

The ACI-TIPI, like the original ACI predictive instrument, provides the ED physician with the 0% to 100% probability that a given patient truly has ACI to supplement the ED triage decision. Its diagnostic performance has been tested in large studies that included ED (3,4) and EMS (5) patients and has been demonstrated to be diagnostically equivalent to the earlier version (3), except for a slightly higher sensitivity for AMI. Thus, clinical use should be comparable to the original ACI predictive instrument (3), with two advantages for clinical use. First, its incorporation into the conventional computerized electrocardiograph allows direct measurement of details of the ECG waveform without the need for physician interpretation, with automatic printing of the ACI probability on the ECG header. Second, its "time insensitivity" makes it valid for retrospective review and assessment of care, as well as for real-time ED clinical care.

Two published early trials have shown impact on the speed and accuracy of ED triage (4,6). Although published only in abstract form, the trial of clinical impact on ED triage decision-making of a 10,689-patient multicenter controlled clinical trial should provide definitive information regarding the impact of the ACI-TIPI. However, because results of abstracts were not considered in arriving at the Working Group's ratings, at this writing, the quality of evidence warrants a C rating and clinical impact a + until rerating once the trial's results are fully published.

The overall results of the Working Group's final ratings of the quality of evidence evaluating this technology and of its ED diagnostic performance and clinical impact are detailed in Table 8.

GOLDMAN CHEST PAIN PROTOCOL

The Goldman computer-based chest pain protocol was developed with the use of a sound methodology. The fact that it was validated

Table 9   Working Group Ratings of Goldman Chest Pain Protocol

ED Diagnostic Performance		ED Clinical Impact	
Quality of Evidence	Accuracy	Quality of Evidence	Impact
A	For AMI: + + + For UAP: NE	B	NK-NE

in a large population that included two university and four community hospitals, with at least two of the hospitals having racially diverse populations, supports its potential utility in a diverse patient population. As the protocol currently stands, its greatest potential benefit would likely be in improving physicians' specificity for AMI and avoidance of triage to the CCU, with attendant cost savings. However, this impact has not been demonstrated in a controlled clinical trial of its use. The only published trial of its impact on care suggests that when it is provided to physicians, there is no impact on care and no change in resource utilization (7).

Given that UAP may be as important as the possibility of AMI with regard to clinical and cost implications, the fact that non–AMI ACI is not addressed by the Goldman protocol is a significant limitation. Moreover, because non–chest pain presentations of ACI (or AMI) are not considered by the protocol, the protocol may well not be applicable for general identification of ACI among all ED patients with symptoms consistent with ACI. Again, its exact clinical value in current practice settings remains to be demonstrated in interventional clinical trials.

The results of the Working Group's final ratings of the quality of evidence evaluating this technology and of its ED diagnostic performance and clinical impact are listed in Table 9.

OTHER COMPUTER-BASED DECISION AIDS

These computer-based decision aids provide examples of a variety of ways to identify patients for CCU admission but have a number of major limitations, especially that they predict AMI rather than ACI and have not yet been demonstrated to be safe and effective in actual use. In addition, there are some concerns about the generalizability and transportability of some of their input variables and, for the neural network model of Baxt (8), concerns about the "black box" and lack of publication of the model to allow testing by others.

Table 10 Working Group Ratings of Other Computer-Based Decision Aids

ED Diagnostic Performance		ED Clinical Impact	
Quality of Evidence	Accuracy	Quality of Evidence	Impact
B	+	NK	NK

Although each of these models has some promise, including very encouraging performance in their preliminary studies, at this point, none can be considered ready for clinical use.

The results of the Working Group's final ratings of the quality of evidence evaluating these technologies and of their ED diagnostic performance and clinical impact are detailed in Table 10.

CREATINE KINASE

Creatine kinase (CK) and CK isoenzyme-cardiac muscle subunit (CK-MB) measurements are traditionally obtained early in the ED course of a patient admitted to the hospital for suspected AMI or ACI. The utility of the assay in the ED as a one-time test is limited because levels do not significantly increase until at least 4 to 6 hours after the onset of AMI. Mass measurements of CK-MB, compared with the older activity analysis, have improved sensitivity and specificity. Improved sensitivity may also be achieved with CK-MB subforms, and these may be more useful in making the diagnosis of AMI in the ED for patients who present early after the onset of symptoms. This is also achieved by the repeated measurements of CK-MB in the ED or the hospital. However, and importantly, CK and CK-MB do not identify patients with UAP, who comprise about half of all patients with ACI.

Despite improvements in the diagnostic performance and practicality of CK and CK-MB assays, there is no controlled clinical impact trial showing that these tests are effective for decisions to send a patient home or to the appropriate level of care of admission for patients with suspected ACI, either as one-time or serial tests. A prospective intervention study, with follow-up of all (including nonadmitted) patients, of the effect of serial CK and CK-MB on patient outcomes is needed before a strategy incorporating CK-MB into medical decisionmaking can be fully evaluated or recommended.

The results of the Working Group's final ratings of the quality

Table 11 Working Group Ratings of CK

| | ED Diagnostic Performance | | ED Clinical Impact | |
	Quality of Evidence	Accuracy	Quality of Evidence	Impact
Single test	A	For AMI: + For UAP: NE	NK	NK
Multiple tests over time	A	For AMI: + + + For UAP: NE	NK	NK

of evidence evaluating this technology and of its ED diagnostic performance and clinical impact are detailed in Table 11.

OTHER BIOCHEMICAL TESTS

Myoglobin, an early marker of AMI, and the cardiac troponins T and I, which are specific for myocyte damage and are late markers, hold promise to improve the identification of patients with AMI and minor myocardial injury. However, the use of new biochemical markers in the ED as a routine measure to improve either the initial triage or therapy of patients with AMI is currently unproven. Although this information may be useful in those hospitals attempting to triage patients between ED holding areas and inpatient beds, the value of their approach needs further bolstering by additional data from carefully controlled studies.

Ultimately, serum protein testing may likely include a panel of multiple markers, which provide a spectrum of information regarding the time of AMI onset. An early sensitive marker such as myoglobin, when combined with CK-MB and troponin-T (increased in the presence of AMI), could provide the clinician with critical information necessary to make decisions in the emergency setting.

The results of the Working Group's final ratings of the quality of evidence evaluating these technologies and of their ED diagnostic performance and clinical impact are detailed in Table 12.

ECHOCARDIOGRAM

Although echocardiography in the ED showed initial promise, it is labor-intensive and insensitive for distinguishing new from old ischemia. Its use in the absence of chest pain appears to be more

Table 12 Working Group Ratings of Other Biochemical Tests

	ED Diagnostic Performance		ED Clinical Impact	
	Quality of Evidence	Accuracy	Quality of Evidence	Impact
Troponin-T and troponin-I	B	For AMI: ++ For UAP: NE	NK	NK
Myoglobin	B	For AMI: + For UAP: NE	NK	NK

accurate in a single study with low numbers for unclear reasons. It can be recommended as an adjunctive test if readily available during atypical chest pain; there are insufficient data demonstrating that it can effectively triage patients in large clinical settings.

Echocardiography is a generally accurate technique, but in the ED setting, when looking for ACI, it still has a false-negative rate that precludes discharging all patients with a negative echo. For the purpose of ruling in or ruling out AMI, echocardiography is unlikely to be done accurately by ED personnel. During hours when expert technicians and interpreters are readily available, echocardiography might improve the accuracy of diagnosis and might thereby lead to a reduction in unnecessary admissions and costs. Beyond the diagnosis of ACI, for those with AMI, additional potentially useful clinical information about complications and hemodynamic status (ejection fraction, pulmonary artery pressure) would also become known, possibly leading to improvements in management and prognosis. Study results that suggest alternative diagnoses that need acute care would also be potentially beneficial.

However, overall, the available investigations to date suggest that even in a *selected* ED population, echocardiography may be reasonably specific but not clearly sufficiently sensitive for either ACI or AMI for this tool to be recommended for ED use. Its role for the overall ED population is even less clear and cannot be recommended without much more information about which patients for whom it should be considered, its diagnostic performance in the usual ED setting, and its safety and effectiveness in this setting when tested in a controlled interventional clinical trial.

The results of the Working Group's final ratings of the quality of evidence evaluating this technology and of its ED diagnostic performance and clinical impact are shown in Table 13.

Table 13 Working Group Ratings of Echocardiogram

ED Diagnostic Performance		ED Clinical Impact	
Quality of Evidence	Accuracy	Quality of Evidence	Impact
B	+	NK	NK

Table 14 Working Group Ratings of Thallium Scanning

ED Diagnostic Performance		ED Clinical Impact	
Quality of Evidence	Accuracy	Quality of Evidence	Impact
C	NK-NE	NK	NK-NE

THALLIUM SCANNING

The use of resting radionuclide imaging for the diagnosis of ACI/AMI in the ED should be restricted to specialized and limited situations in which the clinical triad of history, ECG changes, and enzymatic/laboratory measurements is not available or is unreliable. Such imaging may be helpful, for example, in patients with equivocal chest pain histories and nondiagnostic ECG findings. Thallium-201 is an excellent perfusion tracer, but the available data indicate that the resting scan has relatively poor diagnostic accuracy in the setting of AMI or UAP, with a particularly low specificity. There are also difficulties with isotope availability and tracer redistribution (necessitating imaging within 15 to 20 minutes of injection). Hence thallium-201 does not appear to be an ideal agent for use in the ED management of patients with chest pain.

The results of the Working Group's final ratings of the quality of evidence evaluating this technology and of its ED diagnostic performance and clinical impact are detailed in Table 14.

SESTAMIBI AND OTHER TECHNETIUM-99m PERFUSION AGENTS

The use of radionuclide imaging at rest for the diagnosis of ACI/AMI in the ED should be restricted to specific and limited conditions in which the clinical triad of history, ECG changes, and enzymatic/laboratory measurements is not available or is unreliable. Such imaging may be helpful, for example, in patients with equivocal chest pain histories and nondiagnostic ECG findings. The applicability of this imaging modality depends primarily on logis-

Table 15 Working Group Ratings of Sestamibi and Other Technetium-99 m Perfusion Agents

ED Diagnostic Performance		ED Clinical Impact	
Quality of Evidence	Accuracy	Quality of Evidence	Impact
C	+++	NK	NK

tical issues. Technetium-99m-sestamibi (^{99m}Tc-sestamibi) is an excellent perfusion tracer, with advantageous physical characteristics compared with thallium-201. Its availability, excellent imaging properties, and stable tracer distribution with time make it a practical agent for ED use. Although large-scale trials are lacking, the available data (in relatively small numbers of patients) indicate that ^{99m}Tc-sestamibi is a promising agent for use in the ED evaluation of selected patients with chest pain. Its use to date has been limited to a handful of centers that have studied patients who were judged to be at relatively high risk of having ACI, particularly those having chest pain at the time of the study. It is unclear whether the technique will be of value as a screening test in lower risk ED patients without ongoing chest pain or when used by less experienced interpreters. However, until more evidence is available, it cannot yet be recommended at this stage for general use.

The results of the Working Group's final ratings of the quality of evidence evaluating this technology and of its ED diagnostic performance and clinical impact are shown in Table 15.

CONCLUSIONS AND RECOMMENDATIONS

Summary of Clinical Recommendations Based on Demonstrated Diagnostic Performance and Clinical Impact

Recommendations regarding the use of a technology should be based on both ED diagnostic performance and clinical impact data obtained in high-quality or substantial studies. Of the various diagnostic technologies evaluated in the 14 sections, however, only five met this highly desirable standard of evaluation.

The original ACI predictive instrument was found to be excellent for diagnostic performance (+++) and substantial clinical impact (+++) in a high-quality prospective multicenter trial (A) for both forms of ACI (UAP and AMI). Its accuracy and demonstrated improvement in ED triage make it possible to recommend it for general use in the ED evaluation and triage of patients with symptoms suggestive of ACI. Its main drawback has been that its use requires a programmed calculator or chart, which has been an obstacle to its widespread use. This may be overcome by its successor, the ACI-TIPI, which is incorporated into and reported as part of the header printout on a standard 12-lead ECG.

The second diagnostic technology on which there are studies of both diagnostic performance and clinical impact is the *ACI-TIPI*, although the largest clinical trial of impact is available only in abstract form. It has comparable diagnostic performance (+ + +) to the original ACI predictive instrument based on multicenter prospective studies (A), and the ECG-based ACI-TIPI has ease of use. On the basis of published clinical trials but not including the results of a large prospective trial published to date only in abstract form, its quality of evidence is a C, and clinical impact rating is a +. More definitive recommendations regarding its general use await the full publication of the results of the multicenter trial.

The *prehospital ECG* was found to have good (+ +) diagnostic performance on the basis of evidence from high-quality prospective studies (A). However, this technology was judged to have a small clinical impact (+) on the basis of substantial clinical studies (B). It was the impression of the Working Group, on the basis of these results, that although this technology has promise, it will probably be realized in areas with long EMS transport times. Thus, until more evidence is obtained, its general use cannot be recommended.

The fourth technology for which data are available on both its ED diagnostic performance and clinical impact is the *Goldman chest pain protocol*. An important caveat, however, is that this protocol was designed only for AMI detection and not the more general detection of ACI in the form of UAP. Its diagnostic performance for AMI has been demonstrated to be excellent (+ + +) in multicenter high-quality studies (B). However, in a high-quality prospective study (B), it has not had a demonstrable impact on clinical care (NK/NE), and thus, at this point, its general use cannot be recommended.

The final diagnostic technology, the *ECG exercise stress test*, a different extension of the standard ECG, has also been evaluated to some extent in the ED. Its diagnostic performance for coronary artery disease in this setting has been only modest. Given this, and that its actual impact on triage has received only limited testing, its routine ED use cannot be recommended.

Summary of Clinical Recommendations Based on Demonstrated Diagnostic Performance but Without Data on Clinical Impact

For all but five of the technologies reviewed above there was some published evidence of diagnostic performance but no studies of actual clinical impact (ie, evidence grades were NK for clinical impact). The Working Group strongly advises that, with the exception of the standard 12-lead ECG (see immediately below), diagnostic performance alone is an insufficient basis for recommendation for general use. This is from the long experience of numerous examples of technologies that have excellent or good diagnostic performance but negligible or even negative clinical impact when tested under conditions of actual use (7,9–11).

The *standard 12-lead ECG* has been shown in many studies to have very good, although not perfect, diagnostic performance in the ED. However, despite its key role in the diagnosis of ACI in the ED it has not been demonstrated to have impact on care in the ED setting other than its central role in other technologies such as the ACI predictive instruments described above. In fact, given that the ECG is part of standard ED evaluation, in the view of the Working Group, a trial to demonstrate its impact would be neither necessary nor ethical. Indeed, the 12-lead ECG should be part of the very initial evaluation of any ED or EMS patient with symptoms suggestive of ACI.

Although they have not as of yet been demonstrated to actually improve clinical care in the ED, *blood biochemical tests of myocardial necrosis, particularly CK,* including a variety of assay types and protocols, have undergone prospective testing of their diagnostic performance for the detection of AMI. Available data suggest that the use of a *single CK-MB* test yields performance insufficient for use in ED triage but that the use of *multiple CK-MB* tests over several or more hours has very good diagnostic performance for AMI. Although less complete, the data for *troponin* also suggest that performance of a single test is not satisfactory. The use of multiple tests over time may improve diagnostic performance. The one other biochemical test that has undergone considerable testing is *myoglobin*, but its performance has not yet defined its exact role as an early marker of AMI. Finally, neither myoglobin nor CK detect UAP, which raises the possibility of missing this form of ACI if triage is dependent on such tests. This is one of the reasons that in the absence of prospective trials of the impact of this technology on ED triage (level of admission or discharge), these tests cannot yet be recommended for general ED triage use at this time, although they are very useful for in-hospital care.

Echocardiography, well studied in other settings, has undergone several studies in the ED, which have generally shown modest diagnostic performance for initial ED evaluation. Given this, and that its actual impact on ED care has not been evaluated, this technology cannot be recommended for general ED use at this time.

Radionuclide imaging at rest, although generally used in non-ED settings, has undergone some study of diagnostic performance in the ED. *Thallium scanning* is less appropriate for ED use than sestamibi, has not been evaluated in ED use, and cannot be recommended. *Sestamibi and other technetium-99m perfusion agents* have been studied in the ED setting, and although the overall diagnostic performance of sestamibi has been promising, it has not been sufficiently tested to recommend its general ED use. Whether sestamibi will be found to be more helpful when evaluated for special sub-groups, and when tested for its actual impact on care, remains to be seen. At this point, its general ED use cannot be recommended.

As an extension of the standard ECG, *nonstandard ECG leads* have undergone some limited testing in the ED for detecting ACI, and another prospective trial has been completed. The quality (C) of published data at this point does not provide sufficient evidence of diagnostic utility. In addition, its impact on care has not been tested, and thus nonstandard ECG leads cannot yet be recommended for general use.

Although reported in several case studies in EDs or suggested in a preliminary way in discussions of work done in other settings such as the CCU, *continuous ECG* and *body-surface mapping* have not been tested as to their diagnostic performance in general ED use or for their impact on ED care, and these cannot be recommended for general use at this time.

RECOMMENDATIONS FOR RESEARCH

Although the primary purpose of this report is to provide clinical recommendations, Table 1 makes it clear that there is currently a great lack of research results related to the diagnostic performance and especially the clinical impact of these most important technologies for the emergency evaluation of the most common cause of death in our country. Further diagnostic trials addressing both their accuracy and impact are critical to the NHAAP mission to improve rapidity and effectiveness of care for emergency cardiac patients. Additionally, the evaluation of diagnostic approaches integrating multiple technologies (such as panels of different biochemical markers) or of multiple modalities (such as combining ECG, imaging, and biochemical tests) is needed. In doing this, it will be important to understand the incremental contribution of each modality. In this context, further investigation is needed of the potential utility of computer-based decision aids and analytic programs for integrating and presenting different forms of information.

With more than 6 million patients yearly in this country presenting to the ED with chest pain or analogous symptoms (1,12), with the care of those unnecessarily admitted to cardiac care costing on the order of $3 billion a year (13), and approximately 20,000 ED patients being inappropriately sent home each year (14,15), there is little question that such studies of ways to improve diagnostic and triage performance would be an excellent investment financially and would substantially improve medical care. The Working Group strongly recommends that such studies be supported far more than has been the case to date.

REFERENCES

1. Pozen MW, D'Agostino RB, Selker HP, et al. A predictive instrument to improve coronary-care-unit admission practices in acute ischemic heart disease: a prospective multicenter trial. *N Engl J Med* 1984;310:1273–1278.
2. Pozen MW, D'Agostino RB, Mitchell JB, et al. The usefulness of a predictive instrument to reduce inappropriate admission to the coronary care unit. *Ann Intern Med* 1980;92:238–242.
3. Selker HP, Griffith JL, D'Agostino RB. A tool for judging coronary care unit admission appropriateness, valid for both real-time and retrospective use. A time–insensitive predictive instrument (TIPI) for acute cardiac ischemia: a multicenter study. *Med Care* 1991;29:610–627, erratum 1992;30:188.
4. Cairns CB, Niemann JT, Selker HP, et al. A computerized version of the time-insensitive predictive instrument: use of the Q wave, ST segment, T wave and patient history in the diagnosis of acute myocardial infarction by the computerized ECG. *J Electrocardiol* 1992;24(suppl):S46–S49.
5. Aufderheide TP, Rowlandson I, Lawrence SW, et al. A test of the acute cardiac ischemia time-insensitive predictive instru-

ment (ACI-TIPI) for prehospital use. *Ann Emerg Med* 1996;27: 193–198.

6. Sarasin FP, Reymond JM, Griffith JL, et al. Impact of the acute cardiac ischemia time-insensitive predictive instrument (ACI-TIPI) on the speed of triage decision making for emergency department patients presenting with chest pain: a controlled clinical trial. *J Gen Intern Med* 1994;9:187–194.

7. Lee TH, Pearson SD, Johnson PA, et al. Failure of information as an intervention to modify clinical management: a time-series trial in patients with acute chest pain. *Ann Intern Med* 1995; 122:434–437.

8. Baxt WG. Use of an artificial neural network for the diagnosis of myocardial infarction. *Ann Intern Med* 1991;115:843–888.

9. Selker HP. Coronary care unit triage decision aids: how do we know when they work? *Am J Med* 1989;87:491–493.

10. McCarthy BD, Wong JB, Selker HP. Detecting acute cardiac ischemia in the emergency department: a review of the literature. *J Gen Intern Med* 1990;5:365–373.

11. The SUPPORT Principal Investigators. A controlled trial to improve care for seriously ill hospitalized patients: The Study to Understand Prognosis and Preferences for Outcomes and Risks of Treatments (SUPPORT). *JAMA* 1995;274(20):1591–1598.

12. McCaig L. National Hospital Ambulatory Care Survey: 1992 emergency department summary. *Advanced Data* 1994;245:1–12.

13. Fineberg HV, Scadden D, Goldman L. Care of patients with a low probability of acute myocardial infarction: cost-effectiveness of alternatives to coronary care unit admission. *N Engl J Med* 1984;310:1301–1307.

14. McCarthy BD, Beshansky JR, D'Agostino RB, et al. Missed diagnoses of acute myocardial infarction in the emergency department: results from a multicenter study. *Ann Emerg Med* 1993;22:579–582.

15. Lee TH, Rouan GW, Weisberg MC, et al. Clinical characteristics and natural history of patients with acute myocardial infarction sent home from the emergency room. *Am J Cardiol* 1987;60(4):219–224.

Introduction and Methods

1

As the most common cause of death in this country, acute myocardial infarction (AMI) has deservedly been the subject of substantial efforts of clinicians, scientists, government and other agencies, and the public in efforts to reduce its devastating impact. Although very significant progress continues to be made, the National Heart, Lung, and Blood Institute (NHLBI) of the National Institutes of Health (NIH) recognized the need for a concerted and coordinated effort to reduce mortality and morbidity in this country from AMI and in 1991 initiated the National Heart Attack Alert Program (NHAAP). This ongoing effort, bringing together scientists, clinicians, and NHLBI staff, with the active participation and leadership of a Coordinating Committee that includes representatives of 40 professional organizations, has commissioned a number of working groups to review and make recommendations for physicians and other health care providers about issues related to the rapid recognition and response to patients with symptoms and signs of AMI. Recognizing the central and growing role of diagnostic technologies for AMI and for acute cardiac ischemia (ACI) in general (including both unstable angina pectoris and AMI) in emergency settings, which represent patients' entry points into the health care system, in 1994 the NHAAP Working Group on Evaluation of Technologies for Identifying Acute Cardiac Ischemia in the Emergency Department was formed to assess the utility of diagnostic technologies for ACI/AMI in the emergency department. This report summarizes the Working Group's assessment of the diagnostic performance and impact on care of those technologies. The charge by the NHAAP to the Working Group was to use ACI, rather than AMI, as the diagnostic outcome of interest in the

ED. This reflects the fact that identifying only AMI would miss a large number of ED patients at significant and immediate cardiac risk.

The technologies reviewed address ACI (ie, both AMI and unstable angina pectoris) because this is the condition that must be identified in the treatment of patients with AMI and potential AMI. The review included all such technologies directed at the *diagnosis* of ACI in the ED; methods primarily directed at prognostic or risk stratification of such patients were not included. In this context, to aid the medical community in the use and further evaluation of diagnostic technologies for ACI, this report by the Working Group: 1) comprehensively reviews the important technologies for identifying ACI in the ED setting available at the time of writing and 2) describes the extent to which there are data for each technology that demonstrate its accuracy and effectiveness in actual use in the ED setting. The Working Group was selected to provide expertise in the areas of cardiology, emergency medicine, general internal medicine, family practice, and nursing, as well as in the specific disciplines of metaanalysis and health services research.

WORKING GROUP PROCESS AND METHODS

To accomplish this review, a formal process of review and evaluation of the scientific literature related to these technologies was undertaken based on Medline and related electronic literature searches and supplemented by the panelists' knowledge of the literature and ongoing research. All relevant English-language literature on each technology was reviewed, summarized, analyzed, and reported on independently by three panel members in a process analogous to an NIH Study Section. These reviews were presented in both oral and written format at an initial Working Group meeting, revised and updated by the original authors, and then compiled into a single document by the Working Group cochairs, but without final conclusions and recommendations. This compiled report was reviewed and conclusions and recommendations for each technology were agreed on in a second Working Group meeting. A final update, review, and approval of text and recommendations and conclusions were done before the document was finalized. The report also underwent external review by a broad range of experts who were not members of the Working Group. Because the scientific quality of abstracts cannot be fully evaluated, they were not included in the Working Group's assignment of formal ratings. However, they were included in the discussions of the individual technologies to provide a broad overview.

The written evaluations by the reviewers, subsequent discussions, and compilations followed the following structured format:

I. Summary of Technology
II. Critique
  A. Scientific basis
  B. Clinical practicality
  C. Data from prospective clinical trials in the emergency department setting
    1. Studies of test sensitivity and specificity
    2. Studies of the clinical impact of the test's actual use
  D. Data from other clinical studies
  E. Generalizability to different settings
  F. Applicability to population subgroups, including women and minorities
  G. Cost considerations
  H. Special concerns
  I. Primary advantages
  J. Primary disadvantages
III. Summary and Recommendations

In these evaluations of the clinical data, results were considered applicable to the aims of this report only if they came from work done *in the ED setting*; results coming from other settings (eg, the CCU) were used only if no ED-based data were available. Data from non-ED settings were used with the understanding that they suggest potential utility but do not directly apply to the emergency setting. Assessment of costs was based on the direct costs, when available, of the technology's use. A formal analysis of cost-effectiveness was beyond the scope of this report.

For each technology, studies were formally evaluated and then rated. The *quality of evidence* provided by the relevant studies was rated as A, B, C, or NK, as follows: A, prospective controlled clinical studies of high quality (eg, large multicenter trials with concurrent controls); B, substantial clinical studies; C, limited studies or evidence (eg, case studies, small clinical studies); NK, not known (eg, expert opinion or case reports only).

To validate the Working Group's consensus evidence-based quality rating scoring system, an independent rating of study quality was performed with the use of a detailed, explicit quality rating

3

system of the type typically used in metaanalyses (1,2). Studies of diagnostic test accuracy for ACI/AMI, rather than impact on care, were used for the validity check because there were substantially more studies in this category, which allowed for a better cross-check of agreement of the Working Group's ratings with the more detailed ratings. To provide a relatively homogeneous group for the validity test, the test was done only on those technologies for which there were standard diagnostic categories. A total of 78 studies across eight technologies were scored by the multiitem quality system for comparison with the Working Group's ratings. All these ratings were done by Working Group members, working independently and before designating the Working Group's A, B, C, NK quality ratings at a review meeting.

The explicit quality-assessment form used to evaluate the studies included 26 items, which were divided into four groups for scoring. For each item, the article being rated was rated from zero to a maximum value of 4 points. The scores for the items were summed to provide a score for each study, and these were standardized to a maximum possible of 100 points. The average score for each technology was obtained by averaging the studies within each of the categories assessed.

This evaluation showed a statistically significant Spearman rank correlation of 0.73 between the ratings by the multiitem explicit quality rating system and the rating by the Working Group, supporting the validity of the A, B, C, NK quality rating system used in this report. Moreover, the rank order of the scores followed the Working Group's ratings, again supporting the validity of the A, B, C, NK ratings.

Although primarily intended for the above validation purpose, the multiitem rating system also provided additional useful information about the quality of the studies reviewed. The overall average quality scores derived by the multiitem scoring system were similar to scores assigned with this system to randomized controlled trials of therapies rated over the past 10 years (3). The breakdown analysis by categories provided some insights into the deficiencies of the original reports (1). Perhaps not surprisingly, the weakest area was the actual performance and interpretation of the test. The specific scores over all technologies, by item groups, were as follows: group 1, description of test under investigation and the reference standard used (six items), 83.0; group 2, description of the study population (eight items), 63.9; group 3, description of the performance of tests and interpretation of test results (eight items), 27.1;

group 4, description of statistical analysis and reporting (four items), 45.4.

These results add more detail to the clear implication of the general Working Group ratings of the technologies throughout this report that there is a substantial need for more high-quality assessments of these technologies.

At the second Working Group meeting, on the basis of compiled initial reviews and a consensus process, the panel rated each technology (in addition to the quality ratings described above) for its primary purpose using two distinct metrics: 1) *diagnostic performance*, the accuracy of the technology, measured by sensitivity, specificity, or receiver-operating characteristic curve, for ACI; and 2) *clinical impact*, its demonstrated impact on diagnosis, triage, treatment, or outcome (eg, mortality) when used by clinicians in actual practice.

The *diagnostic performance* of the test and the magnitude of its demonstrated *clinical impact* were rated as $+++$, very accurate/large clinical impact; $++$, moderately accurate/medium impact; $+$, modestly accurate/small impact; NK, not known; NE, not effective.

For example, for prehospital electrocardiography, the quality of evidence for its diagnostic performance was rated as A, and these studies showed moderate accuracy, $++$. For its clinical impact on mortality reduction, the quality of evidence was rated B, and the impact, which was small, was rated as $+$.

The ratings of the Working Group reflect its estimation of the accuracy or impact of the test in actual practice in the ED. These assessments incorporate the quality of the literature, the magnitude or effect size of the reported findings, and considerations of generalizability and feasibility. These ratings take into consideration the text of the reviews but also include a weighting of the evidence by the Working Group. Therefore the text and the ratings, although linked, are sometimes not entirely concordant.

As indicated, in assigning these ratings, each technology was evaluated on the basis of its performance of its *primary* diagnostic purpose of general ED detection, early detection, and detection in specific subgroups. These designations are detailed in Table 1-1.

These technologies all have one of the following as a primary purpose: 1) *The detection of ACI among the general ED population to accurately discriminate patients with ACI from those without ACI among those presenting with symptoms consistent with ACI.* The resting electrocardiogram (ECG) is an example of such a test. 2) *The early identification of ACI, particularly in those with ST-segment elevation due to*

Table 1-1 Primary and Secondary Clinical Purposes of Diagnostic Technologies for ACI

Technology	General ED Detection	Early Detection	Detection in Subgroups
Standard ECG	P	S	S
Prehospital ECG	N	P	N
Continuous 12-lead ECG	N	S	P
Nonstandard ECG leads and body-surface mapping	S	N	P
ECG exercise stress test	N	N	P
Original ACI predictive instrument	P	N	N
ACI-TIPI	P	S	N
Goldman chest pain protocol	P	N	N
Other computer-based decision aids	P	N	N
Creatine kinase	S	S	P
Other biochemical tests	S	S	P
Echocardiogram	N	S	P
Thallium scanning	N	N	P
Sestamibi	N	N	P

P = primary use; **S** = secondary use; **N** = not usual use; **TIPI** = time-insensitive predictive instrument.

AMI. This is the group for whom lifesaving therapy is particularly time-dependent. Technologies for this purpose must have high diagnostic specificity but are intended to provide increased sensitivity for the particular time of interest. An example is the prehospital ECG to detect ST-segment elevation, specifically aimed at providing a positive test for AMI earlier than the ED ECG. 3) *The detection of ACI in certain subgroups.* Such a technology is intended only for certain patients on the basis of specific clinical criteria or preceding test results rather than for the general ED chest pain population. The use of an echocardiogram to confirm an AMI in a patient with tall T waves that might be suggestive of hyperkalemia versus acute ischemia is an example. Biochemical tests that detect AMI but not noninfarction ischemia are another example.

There are other ways to classify these technologies, and in certain circumstances a test may not fit in the category of its usual purpose. Also, some have additional secondary diagnostic roles.

Nonetheless, as a general framework, the primary purposes of the technologies reviewed in this report are summarized in Table 1-1.

Using this framework and the methods outlined above, the following sections report on each technology and the available data supporting its role. The key for interpreting the ratings tables is as follows. For quality-of-evidence rating: A, high-quality clinical studies; B, substantial clinical studies; C, limited studies; NK, not known; NE, not effective. For diagnostic performance and clinical impact rating: +++, very accurate/large clinical impact; ++, moderately accurate/medium impact; +, modestly accurate/small impact; NK, not known; NE, not effective.

The final section summarizes the Working Group's conclusions and recommendations. The executive summary provides a synopsis of methods and results.

REFERENCES

1. Chalmers TC, Smith H Jr, Blackburn B, et al. A method for assessing the quality of a randomized control trial. *Controlled Clin Trials* 1981;2:31–49.
2. Mulrow CD, Linn WD, Gual MK, et al. Assessing quality of a diagnostic test evaluation. *J Gen Intern Med* 1989;4:288–295.
3. Emerson JD, Burdick E, Hoaglin DC, et al. An empirical study of the possible relation of treatment differences to quality scores in controlled randomized clinical trials. *Controlled Clin Trials* 1990;11:339–352.

Standard ECG

2

SUMMARY OF TECHNOLOGY

The primary purpose of the standard ECG is to detect ACI in broad, symptomatic emergency department populations.

The scalar 12-lead ECG is generated by the placement of adherent electrode patches to the surface of the chest and limbs. Each area sampled (a lead) detects voltage, measured in millivolts, and lies in either the frontal or horizontal plane. As myocardial cells depolarize (ie, the outside of the cell changes from positive to negative), an electrical wave phenomenon is generated as depolarization progresses throughout the myocardium.

Normal myocardium depolarizes from endocardium to epicardium and repolarizes from epicardium to endocardium. Ischemic myocardium repolarizes from endocardium to epicardium (ie, opposite of normal) and can therefore write negative, or downward-deflecting, T waves. Likewise, injured myocardium expresses altered electrical activity, which demonstrates elevated ST segments in leads facing the injured area. Leads opposite the injured area can demonstrate ST depression. Necrotic myocardium is electrically neutral and functions as an electrical "window" to the negative charge, which occurs intraventricularly during depolarization. This window in turn allows the electrocardiographic leads facing the necrotic region to "see" a negative charge, which writes a Q wave in those leads facing the necrotic area (1). These electrical phenomena provide the basis for using electrocardiography in the clinical assessment of acute ischemic heart disease.

The inscribed wave forms are interpreted in real time by the emergency physicians and consultants and may be interpreted by a computerized ECG program as well. Such tracings are usually overread (within 24 hours) by physicians credentialed for the "definitive" readings.

CRITIQUE

Scientific Basis

There are several fundamental limitations in the standard ECG. First, it is a single brief sample from a highly varied domain. Because unstable ischemic syndromes have rapidly changing demand and supply characteristics, a single ECG may not adequately represent the entire picture. If a patient with unstable angina is (temporarily) pain free at the time the ECG is obtained, the resulting normal tracing will poorly represent the patient's ischemic myocardium. A tracing taken minutes later may have a very different appearance.

Second, 12-lead electrocardiography is limited because of its lack of perfect detection in areas of the myocardium it samples (2). Small areas of ischemia or infarction may not be detected. Additionally, the conventional leads do not directly examine the right ventricle (3) or the posterior basal or lateral walls very well. AMIs in the distribution of the circumflex artery are likely to have non-diagnostic ECGs (4,5).

Third, some ECG baseline patterns make the ECG tracing difficult or impossible to interpret. These findings include early repolarization, left ventricular hypertrophy, bundle-branch block, and arrhythmias (1). Also, prior Q waves can mask zones of reinfarction, although the presence of any significant abnormality in a patient with chest pain or other related symptoms should generally be considered positive.

Fourth, the waveforms of ECGs are often difficult to interpret, and thus there is much disagreement among readers. Such nonagreement is frequently termed "missed ischemia." This has been studied by Lee and colleagues (6) in their review of patients with AMI who were sent home. The ECGs of such discharged patients tended to have ischemia or infarction not known to be old; 23% of missed diagnoses were due to misread ECGs. These patients were younger, were less likely to have had prior infarct or angina, and had more atypical symptoms.

Jayes et al (7) compared ED physician readings of ECGs with formal interpretations by expert electrocardiographers and calculated sensitivities of 0.59 and 0.64 and specificities of 0.86 and 0.83 for ST-segment and T-wave changes, respectively. McCarthy et al (8) also concluded that 25% of the 20 missed infarcts (of a total of 5,773 patients) were due to incorrect ECG interpretation, a factor emphasized in a review of litigation in missed-AMI cases (9). Correct ECG interpretation by ED physicians is even more critical today because of the need to use thrombolytic agents appropriately in AMI.

Clinical Practicality

The ECG is noninvasive and inexpensive and is universally available in ED settings (10). Additionally, because current protocols for thrombolytic therapy utilize electrocardiographic criteria to determine patient eligibility, ED physicians order ECGs quickly in patients suspected of having acute ischemic heart disease (11). The ECG therefore represents a practical and readily available technology for evaluating patients with acute chest pain.

Data from Prospective Clinical Trials in the ED Setting

Studies of Test Sensitivity and Specificity: Of patients presenting to the ED with acute chest pain, approximately 15% will harbor acute ischemic heart disease (12). The ED ECG, as noted by Lee, is the best single test (13). Another report from Lee et al (14) quantifies the ECG's sensitivity and specificity. This calculation depends, of course, on the criterion chosen for defining normal and abnormal (ie, cutoff for a positive test). If the goal is to diagnose only AMI and select only those ECGs demonstrating probable AMI as positive tests (the most stringent criterion), sensitivity for the ECG (with 95% confidence intervals [CIs]) is 61% (95% CI, 50 to 70) and specificity equals 95% (95% CI, 93 to 97). Positive predictive value for AMI is 73% (95% CI, 64 to 82), and negative predictive value is 92% (95% CI, 90 to 94).

If we use the least stringent criteria for diagnosing AMI (defining ECGs that show any of the following as positive for AMI: nonspecific ST-segment or T-wave changes abnormal but not diagnostic of ischemia; ischemia, strain, or infarction, but changes known to be old; ischemia or strain not known to be old; and probable AMI), we find the following: sensitivity, 99% (95% CI, 94 to 99); specificity, 23% (95% CI, 19 to 27); positive predictive value, 21% (95% CI, 17–25); and negative predictive value, 99% (95% CI, 97 to 100). Using the data from Lee's sensitivity and specificity study (14), the maximum likelihood estimate of the area under the receiver-operating characteristic (ROC) curve for ECG diagnosis of AMI only (not unstable angina) is approximately 0.91.

A report from the Multicenter Chest Pain Study (MCPS) was designed to examine the performance of ED physicians in identifying candidates for thrombolytic therapy (15). Using the positivity criterion of "ST-segment elevation or pathologic Q waves not known to be old," sensitivity for AMI was 41% (95% CI, 33 to 44) and specificity was 98% (95% CI, 97 to 98). Positive predictive value was 76% and negative predictive value was 91%. With the criterion of "ST-segment elevation or depression, or T-wave abnormalities consistent with ischemia or strain, not known to be old," sensitivity was 72% (95% CI, 69 to 75) and specificity was 85% (95% CI, 83 to 86). Positive predictive value was 44% (95% CI, 42 to 46) and negative predictive value was 95% (95% CI, 94 to 96) with this criterion.

These reports suggest that the sensitivity of the ECG depends on how liberally positivity criteria are defined and on whether unstable angina and new-onset angina are included with AMI in defining ACI. A normal ECG appears to have high, but not perfect, negative predictive value for AMI (14). The test can operate with a high true-positive rate but only at the expense of greatly increased false positives.

Studies of the Clinical Impact of the Test's Actual Use: Because evaluation of the ECG is part of the standard of care, there have been no randomized trials of the impact of ECG on the diagnosis of ACI.

Data from Other Clinical Studies

Non-ED studies are not discussed because of the availability of high-quality ED studies.

Generalizability to Different Settings

The MCPS (15) data included patients from a number of large hospital EDs in urban and suburban areas, and the results appear to be generalizable to other similar settings. Also, given that a substantial proportion of ECGs were interpreted by unsupervised house officers, which is less frequently the case now, the generalizability of these data to the current ED situation is not certain. The literature contains no information to indicate how the ECG might function in more rural, community-based settings.

Applicability to Different Subgroups, Including Women and Minorities

The cited studies included both men and women in their evaluations, as well as representative age groups. The published reports do not provide sufficient data subgrouped by minority representation. The incidence of coronary artery disease is variable in different patient populations. Standard ECGs are applicable to all population subgroups, but interpretation may be different. Patients with cocaine-induced chest pain, for example, tend to be younger, with a higher incidence of early repolarization as a normal variant. The interpretation of acute injury must be made with caution in this setting (16). No specific information is available regarding minorities or women separately in the ED.

Cost Considerations

Although the reported studies did not include cost information, the ECG represents an inexpensive and readily available clinical test of approximately $15 to $50 per test.

Special Concerns

The fundamental concern with the ECG is its low sensitivity for AMI (when specificity is high) and for unstable angina. Despite its usefulness, the ECG is insufficiently sensitive to consistently make either diagnosis (17–21). The ECG should not be relied on to make the diagnosis but should rather be included with history and physical examination characteristics to identify patients who appear to be at high risk for ACI. In "rule out AMI" patients, a negative ECG carries an improved short-term prognosis (20,22–25).

Because baseline abnormalities make current evaluation difficult, providing the interpreter with old tracings is of value. Also, sampling should be periodic, not just static. Errors of the following kinds have been documented: 1) not ordering ECGs in younger, atypical patients; and 2) incorrect interpretation, which can be corrected with education aimed at the ED physician. Obtaining a second opinion on an ECG is facilitated by the use of fax transmissions of questionable tracings.

Primary Advantages

Standard ECGs are rapidly available, universal, inexpensive, and "low tech," with reasonable sensitivity and specificity to predict high-risk versus low-risk patients. Accuracy in diagnosis is not perfect but is very high for AMI and is lower for unstable angina.

Primary Disadvantages

Sensitivity is low, as noted above. Additionally, accuracy of the test depends on the skill of the ECG's interpreter. Lee et al (15) found that official ECG interpretations provided higher positive predictive values than those provided by physicians staffing the ED. Another potential problem relates to preexisting ECG changes. Old Q waves, ischemic changes, and conduction defects can impair the interpretation of an ECG for new ischemic findings. Lee et al (26) have demonstrated that when the current ECG tracing demonstrates ischemic findings, "availability of a prior ECG for comparison to determine whether the ECG changes are old or new improves the triage decision by reducing admission of patients without AMI or acute ischemic heart disease without reducing appropriate admissions." Lack of access to old tracings at the ED visit contributes to false-positive triage admission decisions.

SUMMARY AND RECOMMENDATIONS

The ECG represents a safe, readily available, and inexpensive technology for assessing patients with acute chest pain and is central to its evaluation. However, the ECG suffers from imperfect sensitivity and specificity for ACI. When interpreted according to liberal criteria, the ECG operates with relatively high (but not perfect) sensitivity for AMI, at the cost of low specificity. Conversely, when interpreted according to stringent criteria for AMI, sensitivity drops to levels around 50% or below.

The ECG depends on a trained interpreter; less experienced ED interpreters appear to operate at lower positive predictive values than trained interpreters. Additionally, the interpreter frequently cannot tell whether ischemic electrocardiographic changes are new or old because previous tracings are not available or changes such as bundle-branch blocks obscure possible new changes. The ECG's yield is greater during active chest pain, and sensitivity may increase.

In spite of these shortcomings, the standard ECG functions as an integral component of the evaluation of patients with acute chest pain and should continue to be incorporated in strategies that incorporate other clinical characteristics such as historical and physical examination parameters. The ECG is not a perfectly sensitive test, and it should always be considered a supplement to, rather than a substitute for, physician judgment. The Working Group recom-

Table 2-1   Standard ECG

ED Diagnostic Performance		ED Clinical Impact	
Quality of Evidence	Accuracy	Quality of Evidence	Impact
A	++	Standard of care	Standard of care

mends that the ECG continue to be considered the standard of care in the evaluation of chest pain in the ED patient.

The results of the Working Group's final ratings of the quality of evidence evaluating this technology and of its ED diagnostic performance and clinical impact are listed in Table 2-1.

REFERENCES

1. Fisch C. Electrocardiography, exercise stress testing, and ambulatory monitoring. In Kelley WN, ed. *Textbook of Internal Medicine*. Philadelphia: J.B. Lippincott, 1989:305–316.
2. Rude RE, Poole WK, Muller JE, et al. Electrocardiographic and clinical criteria for recognition of acute myocardial infarction based on analysis of 3,697 patients. *Am J Cardiol* 1983; 52:936–942.
3. Lopez-Sendon J, Coma-Canella I, Alcasena S, et al. Electrocardiographic findings in acute right ventricular infarction: sensitivity and specificity of electrocardiographic alterations in right precordial leads V_{4R}, V_{5R}, V_1, V_2, and V_3. *J Am Coll Cardiol* 1985;19(6):1273–1279.
4. Wrenn KD. Protocols in the emergency room evaluation of chest pain: do they fail to diagnose lateral wall myocardial infarction? *J Gen Intern Med* 1987;2:66–67.
5. Nestico PF, Hakki AH, Iskandrian AS, et al. Electrocardiographic diagnosis of posterior myocardial infarction revisited. *J Electrocardiol* 1986;19(1):33–40.
6. Lee TH, Rouan GW, Weisberg MC, et al. Clinical characteristics and natural history of patients with acute myocardial infarction sent home from the emergency room. *Am J Cardiol* 1987;60:219–224.
7. Jayes RL, Larsen GC, Beshansky JR, et al. Physician electrocardiogram reading in the emergency department—accuracy and effect on triage decisions: findings from a multicenter study. *J Gen Intern Med* 1992;7:387–392.

8. McCarthy BD, Beshansky JR, D'Agostino RB, et al. Missed diagnoses of acute myocardial infarction in the emergency department: results from a multicenter study. *Ann Emerg Med* 1993;22:579–582.

9. Rusnak RA, Stair TO, Hansen K, Faston JS. Litigation against the emergency physician: common features in cases of missed myocardial infarction. *Ann Emerg Med* 1989;18:1029–1034.

10. Herr CH. The diagnosis of acute myocardial infarction in the emergency department: part 1. *J Emerg Med* 1992;10:455–461.

11. Muller DW, Topol EJ. Selection of patients with acute myocardial infarction for thrombolytic therapy. *Am Intern Med* 1990; 113:949–960.

12. Lee TH, Weisberg M, Cook EF, et al. Evaluation of creatine kinase and creatine kinase-MB for diagnosing myocardial infarction: clinical impact in the emergency room. *Arch Intern Med* 1987;147:115–121.

13. Lee TH. Chest pain in the emergency department: uncertainty and the test of time. *Mayo Clinic Proc* 1991;66:963–965.

14. Lee TH, Cook EF, Weisberg M, et al. Acute chest pain in the emergency room. Identification and examination of low risk patients. *Arch Intern Med* 1985;145:65–69.

15. Lee TH, Weisberg MC, Brand DA, et al. Candidates for thrombolysis among emergency room patients with acute chest pain. Potential true- and false-positive rates. *Am Intern Med* 1989; 110:957–962.

16. Hedges JR, Kobernick MS. Detection of myocardial ischemia/ infarction in the emergency department patients with chest discomfort. *Emerg Med Clin North Am* 1988;6(2):317–340.

17. Behar S, Schor S, Kariv I, et al. Evaluation of electrocardiogram in emergency room as a decision-making tool. *Chest* 1977;4:486–491.

18. McCarthy BD, Wong JB, Selker HP. Detecting acute cardiac ischemia in the emergency department: a review of the literature. *J Gen Intern Med* 1990;5:365–373.

19. Karlson BW, Herlitz J, Wiklund O, et al. Early prediction of acute myocardial infarction from clinical history, examination and electrocardiogram in the emergency room. *Am J Cardiol* 1991;68:171–175.

20. Bell MR, Montarello JK, Steele PM. Does the emergency room electrocardiogram identify patients with suspected myocardial infarction who are at low risk of acute complications? *Aust N Z J Med* 1990;20:564–569.

21. Sullebarger JT, Greenland P. Myocardial infarction. In Panzer RJ, Black ER, Griner PF, eds. *Diagnostic Strategies for Common Medical Problems*. Philadelphia: American College of Physicians, 1991:55–58.

22. Brush JE, Brand DA, Acampora D, et al. Use of the initial electrocardiogram to predict in-hospital complications of acute myocardial infarction. *N Engl J Med* 1985;312:1137–1141.

23. Fesmire FM, Percy RF, Wears RL, et al. Risk stratification according to the initial electrocardiogram in patients with suspected acute myocardial infarction. *Arch Intern Med* 1989; 149:1294–1297.

24. Zalenski RJ, Sloan EP, Chen EH, et al. The emergency department ECG and immediately life-threatening complications in initially uncomplicated suspected myocardial ischemia. *Ann Emerg Med* 1988;17:221–226.

25. Cohen M, Hawkins L, Greenberg S, et al. Usefulness of ST-segment changes in >/= 2 leads on the emergency room electrocardiogram in either unstable angina pectoris or non–Q-wave myocardial infarction in predicting outcome. *Am J Cardiol* 1991;67:1368–1373.

26. Lee TH, Cook EF, Weisberg MC, et al. Impact of the availability of a prior electrocardiogram on the triage of the patient with acute chest pain. *J Gen Intern Med* 1990;5:381–388.

Prehospital ECG

SUMMARY OF TECHNOLOGY

The primary test purpose for the prehospital ECG is the early detection of AMI with acute ST-segment elevation. One looks to research for answers to two major questions: First, what is the sensitivity/specificity of the prehospital ECG; and second, how much sooner can an appropriate intervention be given for ST-segment elevation AMI detected in the prehospital setting, and does the intervention yield clinical benefit? Direct outcomes (such as mortality) and surrogate outcomes (infarct size on thallium scanning) both can be examined.

Multiple studies have shown the feasibility of performing prehospital 12-lead ECGs (1–12). Diagnostic-quality ECGs can be acquired and successfully transmitted in approximately 70% of prehospital chest pain patients eligible for 12-lead ECGs (3). ECG acquisition increases the time spent at the scene of an emergency an average of 3.9 minutes over control (3). Additionally, there is no difference between the information collected in the prehospital setting and that received by cellular transmission at the base station (1).

The prehospital ECG is obtained in the following manner: 12 leads of analog ECG information are recorded simultaneously for 10 seconds and digitalized at the sampling rate of 250 Hz. After analog-to-digital conversion, the preliminary ECG is printed out in the ambulance. The ECG interpretation is then sent to the hospital by way of cellular telephone through a modem; this takes approximately 20 seconds. Error-free data transmission is ensured by an interactive method of data transfer (1).

The following patients are eligible for prehospital ECGs:

cooperative adult patients with a complaint of chest pain or other symptoms of heart attack, with systolic blood pressure less than 90 mm Hg, and without malignant dysrhythmias (ventricular tachycardia or fibrillation, or second/third-degree atrioventricular block) (4). A prospective evaluation demonstrated that 91.4% of prehospital chest pain patients met these eligibility criteria (3). Three percent to 5% of prehospital patients with complaints of chest pain may be identified as candidates for thrombolytic therapy, which comprises one half or more of all patients receiving thrombolytic therapy (4,6,13).

CRITIQUE

Scientific Basis

Although advances have been made, the available technology that incorporates electrocardiography with defibrillator-monitors is still far from ideal, providing compromises in the format of the 12-lead ECG record, as well as compromising the simple operation of the defibrillator-monitor. The ideal device of the future will provide a standard-format ECG, as well as an integrated defibrillator-monitor (essentially automatic transmission of ECGs to the hospital).

Clinical Practicality

Equipment Choice: First-generation technology combines a monitor, defibrillator, 12-lead ECG capability, and other options such as pacemaking into a single unit that weighs only several pounds more than a standard defibrillator-monitor. This makes prehospital 12-lead acquisition practical for paramedic units. Improvements in size, portability, and choice of hospital reporting formats remain engineering challenges (13).

Paramedic Training: In the United States, paramedics are the primary prehospital health care providers and, in most cases, work under the remote supervision of an emergency physician. Typically these prehospital personnel are required to have more than 1,000 hours of educational training and to participate in regular continuing-education programs. The added paramedic educational requirements to implement prehospital 12-lead electrocardiography is modest, requiring 5 to 7 hours (13).

Data from Prospective Clinical Trials in the Prehospital Setting

Studies of Test Sensitivity and Specificity: In a study of 23 prehospital patients, Grim et al (1) showed that diagnostic-quality ECGs can be recorded by ambulance personnel under the guidance of a hospital-based physician and can be successfully transmitted without error to the receiving hospital. Another prospective study demonstrated improved prehospital diagnostic accuracy for prehospital chest pain patients with a final hospital diagnosis of AMI, angina, and nonischemic chest pain (3). For patients with a final hospital diagnosis of AMI, the specificity of the base physician's prehospital working diagnosis (incorporating both paramedic-acquired history and prehospital 12-lead ECGs) was significantly improved from 68% to 95%, and positive predictive value increased from 33% to 71% when compared with single-lead telemetry (3). When the 12-lead ECG alone was used by base physicians to diagnose AMI, sensitivity was 42% and specificity increased to 99.7% and positive predictive value to 97%, demonstrating that the prehospital 12-lead ECG alone was more accurate in the prehospital diagnosis of AMI patients than the ECG and historical information. Prehospital 12-lead ECGs increased sensitivity from 60% to 79% and increased negative predictive value increased from 57% to 76% for patients with a final hospital diagnosis of angina (3).

The impact that improved prehospital diagnostic accuracy has on patient treatment and outcome for AMI, angina, and nonischemic chest pain patients remains to be fully characterized.

Studies of the Clinical Impact of the Test's Actual Use

Prehospital ECG's Effect on Hospital-Based Time to Treatment: Several studies have demonstrated significant reductions in hospital-based time to treatment with thrombolytic therapy of AMI patients identified before patient arrival with prehospital 12-lead electrocardiography (7,8,10,14). Kereiakes et al (7) demonstrated that the median hospital delay to treatment was 64 minutes for patients transported by private automobile, 55 minutes for patients transported by local ambulance, 50 minutes for patients transported by the emergency medical services (EMS) system with a prehospital ECG obtained but not transmitted to the receiving hospital, and 30 minutes for patients transported by the EMS system who had a 12-lead ECG transmitted from the field. Specialized EMS system transport alone did not facilitate in-hospital initiation of thrombolytic therapy in patients with AMI compared with those brought by local ambulance or private automobile. A significant reduction in hospital delay to treatment was observed only in patients transported by the EMS system who had cellular transmission of a prehospital 12-lead ECG from the field.

Karagounis et al (8) demonstrated a statistically significant 20-minute reduction in time to hospital-based treatment with thrombolytic therapy in AMI patients identified by prehospital 12-lead ECG. Patients with AMI having prehospital 12-lead ECGs were more frequently treated in the ED (rather than in the CCU) and demonstrated a trend toward more rapid ED and CCU treatment.

Prehospital ECG and Prehospital Thrombolysis: The Myocardial Infarction Triage and Intervention (MITI) trial randomized 360 prehospital AMI patients to receive either prehospital or hospital-based thrombolytic therapy (15). Using prehospital 12-lead ECGs and a paramedic contraindication checklist, the MITI trial demonstrated that 353 (98%) of the 360 patients enrolled had subsequent evidence of AMI. Two percent of patients had nondiagnostic abnormalities on the initial ECG. Prehospital identification of patients eligible for thrombolysis by paramedics reduced the hospital treatment time from 60 minutes (for patients not in the study) to 20 minutes (for study patients assigned to begin treatment in the hospital). Because this was not a comparable group by definition, it is only suggestive of the potential benefit of a protocol-driven prehospital thrombolytic program.

The MITI trial also showed that administration of thrombolytics occurred 33 minutes earlier in the prehospital group than in the hospital group, although the investigators found no significant differences overall in mortality, ejection fraction, or infarct size between the prehospital group and the hospital treatment group. Although there was no improvement in outcome associated with initiating treatment before hospital arrival, treatment within 70 minutes of symptom onset was associated with a statistically significant lowered mortality rate of 1.2% (15).

A number of other studies outside the United States have demonstrated that it is possible to accurately identify thrombolytic candidates in the prehospital setting (11,12,16–26).

The Grampion Region Early Anistreplase Trial (22), conducted in northern Scotland, demonstrated a difference of more than 2 hours between prehospital and hospital-based treatment with thrombolytic therapy. This trial demonstrated a statistically significant 50% reduction in 3-month mortality. Furthermore, significantly fewer Q-wave (smaller) myocardial infarctions were seen in patients treated with prehospital thrombolytic therapy than in patients treated in the hospital (22).

The European Myocardial Infarction Project Group reported a randomized trial of prehospital versus hospital thrombolytic therapy (23). In this study, medical personnel (not paramedics) staffed the emergency response units. The two study groups randomized to prehospital or hospital thrombolytic therapies had similar baseline characteristics. The prehospital study group demonstrated a statistically nonsignificant reduction in 30-day mortality in the prehospital group (9.7%) versus the hospital group (11.1%). The cardiac death rate was statistically significantly lower in the prehospital group (8.3% versus 9.8%). Prehospital adverse events such as ventricular fibrillation, shock, hypotension, and bradycardia were more common in the prehospital ECG group than in the hospital-treated group.

In each prehospital thrombolytic trial, prehospital ECGs have led to improved in-hospital diagnosis and shortened treatment times, thereby reducing expected delay associated with usual in-hospital initiation of thrombolytic therapy. These findings, combined with others, suggest that prehospital electrocardiography can improve the diagnostic accuracy of both paramedics and ED physicians in managing patients with chest pain. In addition, when combined with automatic ECG computer interpretation, prehospital ECGs lead to high sensitivity and specificity in differentiating patients with AMI from those with nonspecific chest pain (9,10,27).

The reported potential time savings in prehospital thrombolytic trials range from 30 minutes to more than 2 hours (11,12,15–26,28,29). These studies demonstrate, then, that prehospital treatment with thrombolytic therapy may significantly reduce mortality if the time savings is on the order of 1 hour or more. In rural areas of the United States, where transport times may be exceptionally long, prehospital treatment with thrombolytic therapy may be beneficial. However, it is unknown how many rural EMS systems in the United States have a sophisticated EMS system and an adequate number of thrombolytic candidates to support a prehospital thrombolytic therapy program. Additionally, prehospital treatment of accurately selected thrombolytic candidates may also be the only available method of treating a significant subset of patients within the very early (<70 minutes) time frame.

The Belgian Eminase Prehospital Study (BEPS) also demonstrated significantly more timely thrombolytic therapy for patients treated on the basis of prehospital diagnosis (24). As in the other studies reported above, the BEPS demonstrated shorter times (50 minutes less than in standard hospital care) to thrombolytic administration. However, this trial was not randomized and contained no control group. Also, the prehospital diagnosis and treatment were administered by medical rather than paramedical personnel. Therefore these results might not apply in the United States.

Data from Other Clinical Studies

Studies done outside of the prehospital area are not directly applicable.

Generalizability to Different Settings

The randomized trials reported above appear to be generalizable. The published information derives from trials performed in sophisticated EMS systems. Whether these findings would be obtained in less sophisticated systems remains an open question. Reports from a multicenter effectiveness trial or a prehospital registry would confirm the generalizability of published results of clinical trials.

Applicability to Different Population Subgroups, Including Women and Minorities

The MITI (6,15) reports indicate male predominance in the study population; this might have implications with regard to generalizability (6,15). Additionally, no information appeared regarding minority distribution. The Milwaukee studies (4,5) reported data that indicate essentially equal sex representation; however, the women were significantly older than the men. The other American trials also provided detail regarding minority and sex status insufficient to judge their generalizability (1,10,28,30).

Cost Considerations

Although cost data were not available in the reported literature, a standard defibrillator-monitor with 12-lead ECG capability costs approximately $3,500 to $4,000 more per unit than one without 12-lead ECG capability. An additional $300 investment per electrocardiograph machine is required to purchase a cellular telephone.

Special Concerns

Any EMS system with a prehospital diagnostic strategy should facilitate in-hospital treatment of patients with IV thrombolytic therapy.

Each EMS system should confirm efficient prehospital 12-lead ECG diagnosis and accurate patient candidate identification (13). Prehospital electrocardiographic criteria for the diagnosis of AMI should prioritize the high specificity and a high positive predictive value to minimize false-positive diagnoses (31). Computerized ECG algorithms should be prospectively validated before implementation (13).

In the United States, prehospital 12-lead ECGs should be obtained only under an available verbal or standing written order of a physician. Minimally acceptable written criteria for 12-lead ECG acquisition should be established. Because ECGs are a diagnostic (not therapeutic) modality, application of prehospital 12-lead ECGs in hemodynamically or electrically unstable patients is unwarranted unless the information will be used to triage the patient to a tertiary care facility (13).

Misinterpretation of prehospital 12-lead ECGs may occur. It has been demonstrated that neither computerized algorithms, emergency physicians, nor trained electrocardiographers are 100% accurate in establishing the electrocardiographic diagnosis of AMI. Steps that should be taken to minimize the potential for ECG misinterpretation by ambulance personnel or remote hospital-based physicians include an initial formal educational program in 12-lead ECG interpretation, ongoing educational programs, and 12-lead ECG testing to determine individual competency. Because prehospital 12-lead ECGs must be interpreted in real time without the benefit of comparison with prior 12-lead ECG tracings, personnel should be educated and aware of potential false-positive electrocardiographic patterns, including persistent ST-segment elevation with Q waves after a previous infarction with left ventricular aneurysm, Wolff-Parkinson-White syndrome, left ventricular hypertrophy with strain, early repolarization, hyperkalemia, and left bundle-branch block patterns (13).

Every attempt should be made to correctly identify onscene or transmitted prehospital 12-lead ECGs. Incorrect identification may occur secondary to the simultaneous transmission of two prehospital ECGs from separate ambulances or because an electronically stored ECG is recalled inadvertently rather than the currently acquired record. This problem can be minimized by having ambulance personnel or remote physician interpreters document confirmation of ambulance number, date, time, and the patient's name or initials on the ECG (13).

A central concern of any prehospital diagnostic strategy is the prolongation of paramedic scene time. Average scene delays for 12-lead ECG acquisition are in the range of 4 to 5 minutes (3). It is important to recognize that some individual cases may have scene times significantly longer than the mean. The tangible endpoints of scene time and transport time should be prospectively tabulated after initiation of the program and compared with similar times acquired from retrospective review of hospital records or parallel groups of similar patients in whom prehospital ECGs are not performed. In systems transmitting ECGs, a dedicated telephone line for receiving 12-lead ECG units may avoid a high failed-transmission rate and longer scene time.

Prehospital thrombolytic candidate selection should be driven by a protocol checklist. Historical contraindications checklists should be designed to exclude all potential absolute and relative contraindications, thereby selecting the most obvious patient candidates. Furthermore, a prehospital diagnostic program that has a high specificity and positive predictive value for the diagnosis of AMI and/or thrombolytic candidate selection engenders confidence in the receiving medical community and has the highest likelihood for reducing treatment times (13).

A formal and comprehensive educational program that reviews basic pathophysiology of AMI and myocardial ischemia, ECG application and transmission, and all aspects of the protocol should be administered to prehospital personnel. A formal written protocol for prehospital personnel should be established before program implementation. The protocol should be incorporated into the regional standard EMS system's protocol to prevent interference with standard practice. A qualified individual or committee should be assigned to monitor quality control on an ongoing basis. Continuous feedback of quality-assurance information to prehospital and hospital-based personnel is required to effect constructive change and engender appropriate confidence in the medical community to this approach (13).

EMS systems throughout the United States have varying capabilities. Prioritizing acquisition of 911 within the community, enhanced 911, first-responder defibrillation, and appropriate education of prehospital providers should take precedence over consideration of implementation of prehospital 12-lead ECGs (32).

Primary Advantages

Prehospital 12-lead electrocardiography has been demonstrated to be clinically practical, improve prehospital diagnostic accuracy in chest pain patients, and significantly reduce time to hospital-based treatment with thrombolytic therapy in AMI patients. The prehospital 12-lead ECG would appear to be easily implemented in many established urban paramedic systems and would be a useful adjunct in the rapid triage and treatment of AMI patients. Prehospital diagnosis and treatment of myocardial infarction may be of benefit to many patients provided that the time savings is in the area of 1 hour or more and that the systems to deliver such care can be initiated in a cost-effective manner and implemented properly.

Primary Disadvantages

Implementing a prehospital 12-lead ECG diagnostic strategy represents a significant investment in time, effort, personnel, and cost; there is some concern about the ability of paramedics to maintain these skills over time. Careful attention to quality assurance issues is required. Failed transmission rates may be approximately 10%, and cellular telephone technology currently has no system for prioritizing emergency calls. Prehospital 12-lead electrocardiography does not capture the AMI patients (approximately 50%) who use private transportation to the hospital. The studies also suggest that, using current exclusion criteria, very few chest pain patients would actually receive prehospital thrombolytic therapy. Prehospital 12-lead electrocardiography should be considered only in well-established and relatively sophisticated EMS systems.

SUMMARY AND RECOMMENDATIONS

Studies to date demonstrate that prehospital 12-lead ECG technology is feasible and clinically practical and probably could be implemented in most established urban paramedic systems. *Prehospital identification* of thrombolytic candidates through the use of prehospital 12-lead electrocardiography has been shown in almost every study to significantly reduce hospital-based time to treatment. This time savings is perceived as beneficial but has not, by itself, demonstrated a reduction in mortality. *Prehospital treatment* with

Table 3-1   Prehospital ECG

ED Diagnostic Performance		ED Clinical Impact	
Quality of Evidence	Accuracy	Quality of Evidence	Impact
A	++	B	+

thrombolytic therapy may result in a significant mortality reduction if the time savings is in the area of 1 hour or more. Parallel controlled randomized prospective studies are required to further analyze the cost-benefit issues, additional uses, and ultimate role of prehospital 12-lead electrocardiography.

The results of the Working Group's final ratings of the quality of evidence evaluating this technology and of its ED diagnostic performance and clinical impact are described in Table 3-1.

REFERENCES

1. Grim P, Feldman T, Martin M, et al. Cellular telephone transmission of 12-lead electrocardiograms from ambulance to hospital. *Am J Cardiol* 1987;60:715–720.
2. Aufderheide TP, Hendley GE, Thakur RK, et al. The diagnostic impact of prehospital 12-lead electrocardiography. *Ann Emerg Med* 1990;19:1280–1287.
3. Aufderheide TP, Hendley GE, Woo J, et al. A prospective evaluation of prehospital 12-lead ECG application in chest pain patients. *J Electrocardiol* 1992;24S:8–13.
4. Aufderheide TP, Keelan MH, Hendley GE, et al. Milwaukee Prehospital Chest Pain Project—Phase I: feasibility and accuracy of prehospital thrombolytic candidate selection. *Am J Cardiol* 1992;69:991–996.
5. Aufderheide TP, Haselow WC, Hendley GE, et al. Feasibility of prehospital r-TPA therapy in chest pain patients. *Ann Emerg Med* 1992;21:379–383.
6. Weaver WD, Eisenberg MS, Martin JS, et al. Myocardial Infarction Triage and Intervention Project—Phase I: patient characteristics and feasibility of prehospital initiation of thrombolytic therapy. *J Am Coll Cardiol* 1990;15:925–931.
7. Kereiakes DJ, Gibler WB, Martin LH, et al. Relative importance of emergency medical system transport and the prehospital electrocardiogram on reducing hospital time delay to therapy for acute myocardial infarction: a preliminary report from the Cincinnati Heart Project. *Am Heart J* 1992;23:835–840.
8. Karagounis L, Ipsen SK, Jessop MR, et al. Impact of field-transmitted electrocardiography on time to in-hospital thrombolytic therapy in acute myocardial infarction. *Am J Cardiol* 1990;66:786–791.
9. O'Rourke MF, Cook A, Carroll G, et al. Accuracy of a portable

interpretive ECG machine in diagnosis of acute evolving myocardial infarction. *Aust N Z J Med* 1992;22:9–13.

10. Foster DB, Dufendach JH, Barkdoll CM, et al. Prehospital recognition of AMI using independent nurse/paramedic 12-lead ECG evaluation: impact on in-hospital times to thrombolysis in a rural community hospital. *Am J Emerg Med* 1994; 12(1):25–31.

11. Koren G, Weiss AT, Ben-David AT, et al. Prevention of myocardial damage in acute myocardial ischemia by earlier treatment with intravenous streptokinase. *N Eng J Med* 1985;313: 1384–1389.

12. Fine DG, Weiss AT, Sapoznikov D, et al. Importance of early initiation of intravenous streptokinase therapy for acute myocardial infarction. *Am J Cardiol* 1986;58(6):411–417.

13. Aufderheide TP, Kereiakes DJ, Weaver WD, et al. Planning, implementation, and process monitoring for prehospital 12-lead ECG diagnostic programs. *Prehospital and Disaster Medicine* 1996;11(3):162–171.

14. Aufderheide TP, Lawrence SW, Hall KN, et al. Prehospital 12-lead electrocardiograms reduce hospital-based time to treatment in thrombolytic candidates (abstract). *Acad Emerg Med* 1994;1(2):A13–A14.

15. Weaver WD, Cerqueira M, Hallstrom AP, et al. Prehospital-initiated vs hospital-initiated thrombolytic therapy. The Myocardial Infarction and Intervention Trial. *JAMA* 1993;270:1211–1216.

16. Bippus P, Storch W, Andresen D, et al. Thrombolysis started at home in acute myocardial infarction: feasibility and time-gain. *Circulation* 1987;76(suppl IV):IV–122.

17. Holmberg S, Hjalmarson A, Swedberg K, et al. Very early thrombolysis therapy in suspected acute myocardial infarction. *Am J Cardiol* 1990;65:401–407.

18. Oemrawsingh P, Bosker H, Vanderlaarse A, et al. Early reperfusion by initiation of intravenous streptokinase prior to ambulance transport. *Circulation* 1988;78(suppl II):II–110.

19. Castaigne A, Herve C, Duval-Moulin A, et al. Prehospital use of APSAC: results of placebo-controlled study. *Am J Cardiol* 1989;64(2):30A–33A.

20. Bossaert L, Demey H, Colemont L, et al. Prehospital thrombolytic treatment of acute myocardial infarction with an isolated plasminogen streptokinase activator complex. *Crit Care Med* 1988;16:823–830.

21. Rawles J, on behalf of the GREAT Group. Halving of mortality at 1 year by domiciliary thrombolysis in the Grampian Region Early Anistreplase Trial (GREAT). *J Am Coll Cardiol* 1994;23:1–5.
22. Roth A, Barbash G, Hod H, et al. Should thrombolytic therapy be administered in the mobile intensive care unit in patients with evolving myocardial infarction? *J Am Coll Cardiol* 1990; 14:932–936.
23. The European Myocardial Infarction Project Group. Prehospital thrombolytic therapy in patients with suspected acute myocardial infarction. *N Engl J Med* 1993;329:383–389.
24. BEPS Collaborative Group. Prehospital thrombolysis in acute myocardial infarction: the Belgian Eminase Prehospital Study (BEPS). *Eur Heart J* 1991;12:965–967.
25. Risenfors M, Gustavsson G, Ekstrom L, et al. Prehospital thrombolysis in suspected acute myocardial infarction: results from the TEAHAT Study. *J Intern Med* 1991;229(suppl 1):401–407.
26. Weiss A, Fine D, Applebaum D, et al. Prehospital coronary thrombolysis, a new strategy in acute myocardial infarction. *Chest* 1987;92:124–128.
27. Kudenchuk PJ, Ho MT, Weaver WD, et al. Accuracy of computer-interpreted electrocardiography in selecting patients for thrombolytic therapy. *J Am Coll Cardiol* 1991;17:1486–1491.
28. Gibler WB, Kereiakes DJ, Dean EN, et al. Prehospital diagnosis and treatment of acute myocardial infarction: a North-South perspective. *Am Heart J* 1991;121:1–11.
29. Aufderheide TP, Keelan MH, Lawrence SH, et al. The Milwaukee Prehospital Chest Pain Project: Phase II. A randomized trial of pre-hospital versus hospital-based thrombolytic therapy for acute myocardial infarction patients (abstract). *Acad Emerg Med* 1994;1(2):A8.
30. Kereiakes DJ, Weaver WD, Anderson JL, et al. Time delays in the diagnosis and treatment of acute myocardial infarction: a tale of eight cities. Report from the Prehospital Study Group and the Cincinnati Heart Project. *Am Heart J* 1990;120:773–780.
31. Otto LA, Aufderheide TP. Evaluation of ST segment elevation criteria for the prehospital electrocardiographic diagnosis of acute myocardial infarction. *Ann Emerg Med* 1994;23:17–24.
32. Ornato JP, Aufderheide TP, Wynn J, et al. Working group report: present and future prehospital management. In LaRosa JH,

Horan MJ, Passamani ER, eds. *Proceedings of the National Heart, Lung, and Blood Institute Symposium on Rapid Identification and Treatment of Acute Myocardial Infarction.* Bethesda, MD: US Department of Health and Human Services, Public Health Service, National Institutes of Health, 1991;139–141.

Continuous 12-Lead ECG

4

SUMMARY OF TECHNOLOGY

In the context of the mission of the National Heart Attack Alert Program, continuous electrocardiography could address two purposes. First, it could aid in the early detection of potential candidates for thrombolysis or angioplasty while being monitored in the emergency department. This may occur in patients with suspected AMI whose initial ECG is nonspecific but whose second ECG has at least 0.1 mV of ST-segment elevation in two contiguous leads. Second, in subgroups of ED patients it could improve the diagnosis of ACI by detecting ST-segment changes that confirm the diagnosis of unstable angina or non–Q-wave AMI. It is outside of the scope of this report to consider the role of continuous ECG in the detection of vessel patency in thrombolytic-treated patients.

A typical instrument for continuous ST-segment monitoring is microprocessor controlled and fully programmable (1). In the default settings, it continuously acquires a new 12-lead ECG every 20 seconds and analyzes the ST segments. The ST segments are measured at the J point plus 60 milliseconds. The magnitude of the ST segments is saved for later retrieval. The limb leads are positioned on the torso for optimal noise reduction (the precordial leads are placed in the standard position). The initial ECG is defined as the pretrigger ECG. If ST-segment elevation or depression of 0.2 mV or greater occurs in a single lead or 0.1 mV in two leads compared with the pretrigger ECG, the device enters a potential alarm state. If four sequential ECGs have met the threshold criteria, then an alarm sounds and a 12-lead ECG is printed for physician review. This ECG then becomes the new pretrigger ECG for future ST-segment comparisons. Typically, a 12-lead ECG is saved every 20 minutes, as well as any alarm ECGs. Options allow one to save an ECG at any time for later review. During the monitoring process, the physician can print any three ECGs for comparison purposes. One can also print two-dimensional graphs of ST-segment trends (magnitude versus time) for the 12 individual leads or the average ST-segment magnitudes for the four regional groupings: anterior (V_1–V_3), inferior (II, III, aVF), low lateral (V_4–V_6), and high lateral (I, aVL). At the termination of the monitoring session, summary statistics are printed that consist of the monitoring interval, the maximum ST-segment depression and elevation for the frontal and precordial leads, the number of ECGs stored, and the number of alarms that sounded.

A current limitation is that such devices do not automatically detect changes other than ST-segment displacement that are suggestive of AMI such as loss of R-wave progression or changes suggestive of ischemia such as new T-wave inversions. Also, ST-segment changes below the specified voltage thresholds will not be automatically detected. These limitations, however, can be overcome if the physician operator manually prints and reviews serial ECGs.

CRITIQUE
Scientific Basis

The practice of monitoring dysrhythmias in suspected cardiac patients became the standard of care when electrical and chemical defibrillation demonstrated the potential to terminate dysrhythmias. Similarly, with the advent of specific proven modalities to treat both AMI (with thrombolytics or angioplasty) and myocardial ischemia (with anticoagulants, vasodilators, circulation support devices, and angioplasty), there are sound reasons to evaluate and test the continuous 12-lead ECG.

In patients at risk, waiting for the clinical detection of dysrhythmias (eg, syncope) is unwise. It also may be unwise to rely on clinical manifestations of ischemia in patients at risk. Changes in coronary blood flow and injury patterns subsequently detected by ECG are very variable and often silent (1–3). Monitoring these by clinical indications only may be poorly sensitive for detecting these ECG changes. Theoretically, continuous 12-lead ECGs have a much better chance of capturing these changes (2,4–13). Performing ECGs only when patients complain of pain, the current practice, may result in inadequate ECG surveillance for a number of reasons: Patients' symptoms do not reflect the full ischemic burden, patients probably underreport chest pain symptoms, and even when an emergency nurse or physician receives a report of increased or recurrent pain, by the time the 12-lead ECG is performed the symptoms and the concomitant ECG findings may be absent in some patients (1–3,14–17).

These physiologic, patient behavior, and logistic issues present a sound rationale for the evaluation of continuous ECGs in the ED. Nonetheless, there are potential difficulties with this technology. Although unequivocal ECG changes accompanied by clinical findings would be clearly useful, a host of other ST-segment displacements will be detected in the resting asymptomatic patients. The use of asymptomatic ST-segment depression or even elevation in that setting is both a diagnostic and a therapeutic unknown.

Because approximately 50% of the patients with chest pain and AMI present to the ED without ST-segment elevation, and in-hospital electrocardiographic evidence of transmural infarction develops in nearly 20% of these patients, continuous serial ECGs with ST-segment trend monitoring may identify the patient population most likely to benefit from rapid interventions after detection of electrocardiographic criteria diagnostic for AMI (18).

In summary, the advantages of continuous 12-lead electrocardiographic monitoring in an ED setting include detection of silent myocardial ischemia and infarction and detection of symptomatic individuals otherwise missed who receive a nonscheduled ECG only after complaints of pain have subsided. ST-segment trend monitoring may provide the earliest evidence of coronary occlusion in patients presenting with preinfarction angina (18).

Clinical Practicality

Current technology makes 12-lead ST-segment monitoring possible with a wall-mounted device or a portable device suitable for transportation (18,19). ST-segment monitoring can be initiated rapidly before or immediately after the onset of symptoms and can be continued for as long as the patient is at bed rest. Clinical trials have demonstrated that this technology can be initiated in a timely and practical fashion (15,18,20,21). The information is printed in typical 12-lead ECG format and can usually be interpreted without difficulty (18,22). Continuous 12-lead ST-segment monitoring may be feasible in an ambulance or ambulance/helicopter setting.

Cardiac electrical signals are transferred from the patient to the 12-lead. ECG/ST-segment trends are monitored through cables attached to 10 stress-type electrodes (4 limb, 6 precordia). The constant tethering of the patient by cable to the electrocardiograph can be a source of patient discomfort, particularly if the observation period is prolonged.

The continuous 12-lead ECG/ST-segment trend-monitoring equipment is small (approximately 4 inches high, 12 inches wide, and 12 inches long; total weight, 10 pounds), allowing bedside placement and transportability. Data can be obtained in a paper format or transferred by digital signal through a land line to a standard cathode ray tube computer/monitor for further data analyses.

Data From Prospective Clinical Trials in the ED Setting

Studies of Test Sensitivity and Specificity: There are no data from prospective ED trials of continuous ECG to assess sensitivity and specificity. In a retrospective study, Gibler et al (23) used ECG/ST-segment trend monitoring to monitor 1,010 patients in a chest pain evaluation and treatment program located in the ED. Of 52 patients with cardiac disease, 11 had evidence of ischemia or evolving AMI by ST-segment trend monitoring. Because this population had a low prevalence of acute ischemic coronary syndrome, it is hypothesized that such a monitoring device may actually demonstrate a higher utility in a population with greater disease prevalence.

In earlier trials, Gibler et al (18) evaluated 86 patients with chest discomfort admitted to a heart ED program. Eighteen patients (20.9%) had cardiac diagnoses on discharge from the hospital after in-hospital evaluations for ACI. Serial 12-lead ECGs with ST-segment trend monitoring detected 7 of 18 patients (39%) with a final cardiac diagnosis consistent with ACI. Ten patients had ST-segment trend monitoring with positive results, but hospitalization revealed a non-cardiac cause of their chest discomfort. Thus the positive predictive value was less than 50%, meaning that there were more false positives than true positives.

Studies of the Clinical Impact of the Test's Actual Use: There are no studies, only case reports, of clinical impact.

Two recent case reports describe potential advantages of continuous 12-lead ST-segment monitoring in the ED setting. Fu et al (24) describe a case of a 48-year-old man in whom AMI was detected by continuous ST-segment monitoring while the patient was asymptomatic. In this case, the use of continuous 12-lead ST-segment monitoring allowed for early therapeutic intervention, including rapid infusion of thrombolytic therapy. Fesmire and

Bardoner (3) describe a patient with AMI who demonstrated transient, silent ST-segment elevations and depressions preceding cardiac arrest. The authors contend that it may be possible to identify continuous 12-lead ST-segment patterns that identify patients at high risk for sudden death and AMI.

Data from Other Clinical Studies

In a related study of serial ECGs, Hedges et al (25) evaluated 261 ED patients with chest discomfort, independently analyzing the accuracy of serial creatine kinase isoenzyme–cardiac muscle subunit (CK-MB) measurements and serial ECGs (defined as ECGs acquired at presentation and 3 to 4 hours after presentation). Sensitivity of serial ECG changes versus serial CK-MB levels diagnostic of AMI was 39% versus 68%; specificity was 88% versus 95%. Two of 261 patients (0.8%) without initial ST-segment elevation were found to have ST-segment elevation on reevaluation and became thrombolytic candidates. The authors concluded that serial changes in ECGs during a 3- to 4-hour interval were associated with the diagnosis of AMI but were infrequent and less accurate than serial CK-MB levels obtained for the same interval.

Relevant to the first test purpose, that of detecting new ST-segment elevation AMI, Krucoff and colleagues (10,11,16,19–22) have conducted a number of studies that evaluated continuous ST-segment monitoring in a CCU setting. Using two- to three-lead ST-segment Holter recordings, investigators found that achievement of ST-segment steady state before steptokinase infusion was 100% sensitive and 100% specific for subtotal rather than total occlusion. These data support the contention that continuous ST-segment monitoring combines good sensitivity and specificity in noninvasively detecting infarct vessel patency during an AMI. However, such studies have not been published for an ED cohort of high-risk patients.

The number of leads that should be continuously monitored is open to question. Data from the balloon angioplasty setting (15) suggest that only 4 of 12 leads (V2, V3, III, V5) were needed to achieve 100% sensitivity in detecting ST-segment elevation or depression of at least 0.1 mV in one lead during balloon inflation.

Outside the ED setting, there are numerous reports regarding ischemia detection by continuous monitoring of selected ECG leads (10,11,14,16,19–22,26–28). Studies generally have found that ECGs in the early hospital and outpatient settings are predictive of a significant increase in cardiac events (15,28–30). Johnson et al (30) found that in a group of patients with clinically unstable angina pectoris, transient ST-segment displacement was associated with higher rates of three-vessel coronary artery disease and poor prognosis over a 3-month follow-up period. However, regarding specificity, Eggeling et al (29) reported Holter monitoring revealed episodes of 0.1 mV of downsloping ST-segment depression of at least 1 minute's duration in nondiseased patients, so in this report specificity was not found to be 100%.

Gottlieb (31) considers ST-segment monitoring an alternative for those unable to perform exercise testing. Holter-like devices with continuous ST-segment monitoring capability in one to three leads have been used in an ambulatory setting to diagnose silent and symptomatic ischemia and in the inpatient setting to diagnose ischemia in the anesthetized postsurgical patient and in post-thrombolytic patients. Essen et al (32) used monitoring in three to eight leads continuously in conjunction with precordial mapping to increase the sensitivity of detecting ischemia or injury in patients undergoing thrombolytic therapy.

Generalizability to Different Settings

Because there are no ED cohort studies on the use of continuous ECG, the issues of external validity cannot be assessed.

Applicability to Population Subgroups, Including Women and Minorities

There are no applicable reports.

Cost Considerations

Technology is currently evolving, but continuous ECG may represent substantial financial investment along with a combined commitment from the departments of emergency medicine and cardiology to this new approach. Monitors cost approximately $8,000 per bed; central monitor stations cost approximately $15,000.

Special Concerns

Although one lead is usually sufficient for arrhythmia monitoring, it is currently unclear how many leads are needed for ischemia or injury monitoring. Angioplasty data suggest that only four leads are needed to detect ischemia in that setting (15). Patient comfort is another concern that may affect results. Patients often experience discomfort from being tethered to a cable, and baseline artifact from patient movement or cable damage may result in an inaccurate interpretation.

Primary Advantages

In the ED, continuous 12-lead ECG monitoring may provide the earliest evidence of coronary occlusion in patients presenting with preinfarction angina and may detect silent myocardial ischemia and AMI that might otherwise remain undetected. It may thus increase the sensitivity of ECG testing for injury patterns leading to the identification of more potential thrombolytic candidates. It may also help confirm the diagnosis of ACI in chest pain patients undergoing evaluation in the ED. In ED patients with nondiagnostic 12-lead ECGs, continuous ECG monitoring may raise the sensitivity of the ECG, which may assist in safely discharging patients with nonischemic causes of chest pain. Because it is identical to standard ECG testing, diffusion should be straightforward.

Primary Disadvantages

The benefits and costs are unknown. If ECG findings detected by continuous ECG have low specificity, they may lead to unnecessary hospitalizations. However, preliminary data do not suggest that this is a large problem (23). T waves and ST segments may be labile as a result of hyperventilation, patient movement, or posture, requiring overreading by the treating clinician. The increased burden on understaffed EDs required to continuously monitor and care for patients with continuous 12-lead ECGs may be significant.

SUMMARY AND RECOMMENDATIONS

There have been no well-designed large randomized prospective ED or CCU studies evaluating this technology. Cost-benefit analysis of this technology has not been accomplished. Although ED ST-segment monitoring holds the potential to detect silent myocardial ischemia and infarction, reduce missed ischemic diagnoses, and provide the earliest evidence for coronary occlusion in patients pre-

Table 4-1 Continuous 12-Lead ECG

ED Diagnostic Performance		ED Clinical Impact	
Quality of Evidence	Accuracy	Quality of Evidence	Impact
NK	NK	NK	NK

senting with preinfarction angina, larger prospective studies are required to make this assessment.

The results of the Working Group's final ratings of the quality of evidence evaluating this technology and of its ED diagnostic performance and clinical impact are shown in Table 4-1.

REFERENCES

1. Fesmire FM, Smith EE. Continuous 12-lead electrocardiograph monitoring in the emergency department. *Am J Emerg Med* 1993;11:54–60.
2. McHugh P, Gill NP, Wyld R, et al. Continuous ambulatory ECG monitoring in the preoperative period: relationship of preoperative status and outcome. *Br J Anaesth* 1991;66:285–291.
3. Fesmire FM, Bardoner JB. ST-segment instability preceding simultaneous cardiac arrest and AMI in a patient undergoing continuous 12-lead ECG monitoring. *Am J Emerg Med* 1994; 12:69–76.
4. Wilcox I, Freedman BS, Li J, et al. Comparison of exercise stress testing with ambulatory electrocardiographic monitoring in the detection of myocardial ischemia after unstable angina pectoris. *Am J Cardiol* 1991;67:89–91.
5. Stern S, Tzivoni D. Early detection of silent ischemic heart disease by 24-hour electrocardiographic monitoring of active subjects. *Br Heart J* 1974;36:481–486.
6. Turitto G, Caref EB, Zanchi E, et al. Spontaneous myocardial ischemia and the signal-averaged electrocardiogram. *Am J Cardiol* 1991;67:676–680.
7. Feldman RL. Ambulatory electrocardiographic monitoring: the test for ischemia in 1988? *Ann Intern Med* 1988;109:608–610.
8. Knight AA, Hollenberg M, London MJ, et al. Perioperative myocardial ischemia: importance of preoperative ischemic pattern. *Anesthesiology* 1988;68:681–688.
9. Knight AA, Hollenberg M, London MJ, et al. Myocardial ischemia in patients awaiting coronary artery bypass grafting. *Am Heart J* 1989;117:1189–1196.
10. Krucoff MW, Green CE, Satler LF, et al. Noninvasive detection of coronary artery patency using continuous ST segment monitoring. *Am J Cardiol* 1986;57:916–922.
11. Krucoff MW, Parente AR, Bottner RK, et al. Stability of multilead ST-segment fingerprints over time after percutaneous

transluminal coronary angioplasty and its usefulness in detecting reocclusion. *Am J Cardiol* 1988;61:1232–1237.

12. Hackett D, Davies G, Chierchia S, et al. Intermittent coronary occlusion in acute myocardial infarction: value of combined thrombolytic and vasodilator therapy. *N Engl J Med* 1987;317: 1055–1059.

13. Hogg KJ, Hornung RS, Howie CA, et al. Electrocardiographic prediction of coronary artery patency after thrombolytic treatment in acute myocardial infarction: use of the ST segment as a non–invasive marker. *Br Heart J* 1988;60:275–280.

14. Califf RM, O'Neil W, Stack RS, et al. Failure of simple clinical measurements to predict perfusion status after intravenous thrombolysis. *Ann Intern Med* 1988;108:658–662.

15. Mizutani M, Freedman S, Barns E. ST monitoring for myocardial ischemia during and after coronary angioplasty. *Am J Cardiol* 1990;66:389–393.

16. Krucoff M. Identification of high–risk patients with silent myocardial ischemia after percutaneous transluminal coronary angioplasty by multilead monitoring. *Am J Cardiol* 1988;61(12): 29F–35F.

17. Hoberg E, Schwarz F, Voggenreiter U, et al. Holter monitoring before, during, and after percutaneous transluminal coronary angioplasty for evaluation of high–resolution trend recordings of leads CM_5 and CC_5 for ST-segment analysis. *Am J Cardiol* 1987;60:796–800.

18. Gibler WB, Sayre MR, Levy RC, et al. Serial 12–lead electro-cardiographic monitoring in patients presenting to the emergency department with chest pain. *J Electrocardiol* 1994;26S: 238–243.

19. Krucoff MW, Wagner NB, Poper JE, et al. The portable programmable microprocessor-driven real-time 12-lead electrocardiographic monitor: a preliminary report of a new device for the noninvasive detection of successful reperfusion or silent coronary reocclusion. *Am J Cardiol* 1990;65:143–148.

20. Krucoff MW, Croll MA, Pope JE, et al. Continuously updated 12-lead ST segment recovery analysis for myocardial infarct artery patency assessment and its correlation with multiple simultaneous early angiographic observations. *Am J Cardiol* 1993;71:145–151.

21. Krucoff MW, Croll MA, Pope JE, et al. Continuous 12-lead ST-segment recovery analysis in the TAMI 7 study. *Circulation* 1993;88:437–446.

22. Krucoff MW, Croll MA, Pope JE, et al. Heuristic and logistic principles of ST-segment interpretation in the time domain. *J Electrocardiol* 1990;23S:6–10.

23. Gibler WB, Runyon JP, Levy RC, et al. A rapid diagnostic and treatment center for patients with chest pain in the emergency department. *Ann Emerg Med* 1995;25:1–8.

24. Fu GY, Joseph AJ, Antalis G. Application of continuous ST-segment monitoring in the detection of silent myocardial ischemia. *Ann Emerg Med* 1994;23:1113–1115.

25. Hedges JR, Young GP, Henkel GF, et al. Serial ECGs are less accurate than serial CK-MB results for emergency department diagnosis of myocardial infarction. *Ann Emerg Med* 1992;21: 1445–1450.

26. Veldkamp RF, Bengtson JR, Sawchak ST, et al. Evolution of an automated ST-segment analysis program for dynamic real-time non-invasive detection of coronary occlusion and reperfusion. *J Electrocardiol* 1992;25(suppl):182–187.

27. Wilcox I, Breedman S, Kelly D, et al. Clinical significance of silent ischemia in unstable angina pectoris. *Am J Cardiol* 1990; 65:1313–1316.

28. Hedblad B, Juul-Moller S, Svensson K. Increased mortality in men with ST segment depression during 24 hour ambulatory long-term ECG recording. *Eur Heart J* 1989;10:149–158.

29. Eggeling T, Gunther H, Teris-Mueller I, et al. ST segment changes in healthy volunteers during Holter monitoring and exercise stress test. *Eur Heart J* 1988;9(suppl N):61–64.

30. Johnson S, Mauritson D, Winniford M. Continuous ECG monitoring in patients with unstable angina pectoris. *Am Heart J* 1982;103:4–12.

31. Gottlieb SO. Preoperative myocardial ischemia and infarction. Detection of myocardial ischemia using continuous ECG (abstract). *Int Anesthesiol Clin* 1992;30(1):19–30.

32. von Essen R, Schmidt W, Uebis R, et al. Myocardial infarction and thrombolysis: electrocardiographic short term and long term results using precordial mapping. *Br Heart J* 1985;54:6–10.

Nonstandard ECG Leads and Body-Surface Mapping

5

SUMMARY OF TECHNOLOGY

The standard 12-lead ECG is a less-than-perfect predictor of AMI. The sensitivity of ST-segment elevation for AMI is approximately 50% (1), and as many as 30% of AMI patients have nonspecific or normal ECGs. One of the explanations offered for these limitations is that the 12-lead ECG poorly detects posterior wall (2) and right ventricular infarction (RVI). These areas of the myocardium are not directly interrogated by standard leads but are assessed by posterior leads V_7, V_8, and V_9 and right-sided leads V_{4R}, V_{5R}, and V_{6R} (3).

Posterior AMI is one of the most commonly missed ECG findings, and this may be explained by the lack of direct ECG examination (4). In their study, Seyal and Swiryn (5) found that 6% of infarctions (13 of 250) are isolated to the posterior basal surface of the left ventricle. In another study, about half of the patients with isolated circumflex lesions displayed the "RV" (tall R wave in V_1) pattern of posterior AMI (6). RVI occurs in approximately 40% of inferior AMIs and about 4% of the time as an isolated entity (7). ST-segment elevation in lead V_{4R} in the setting of inferior AMI is a sensitive and specific marker of RVI (7–11).

Posterior and right-sided leads are acquired using the same electrocardiograph as standard leads. For right-sided leads, the lead placement is just the reverse of standard left-sided leads (ie, mid-clavicular line, fifth intercostal space for V_{4R}, anterior axillary line for V_{5R}, and midaxillary line for V_{6R}). Posterior leads continue in the same horizontal plane as the precordial leads (ie, fifth intercostal space, but continue on to the posterior axillary line for V_7, midscapular line for V_8, and paraspinal for V_9).

Body-surface mapping uses multiple (approximately 120) leads over the entire torso (anterior and posterior) to record repolarization voltage changes to optimally discriminate between AMI and non-AMI. Body-surface mapping has been used to determine the location and size of the infarcted area in AMI, assess efficacy of interventions designed to limit infarct size, and improve diagnostic ability compared with that of standard 12-lead ECG (12–17). Body-surface mapping techniques have been applied to highly selected patient populations and use up to 87 leads with specialized interpretation. This technology has been used primarily as a valuable research tool to provide semiquantitative and quantitative data regarding infarct location and size, but it may be more widely used as software interfaces improve (12–15,17).

Chaos analysis detects disorder (rather than maximum displacement) in the voltage signal characteristics produced by ischemic myocardium and compares this to characteristics produced by normal myocardium. The program that detects this is a proprietary product. It is composed of a patient interface, signal preprocessor, signal storage, signal analysis, and data–display modules (18). The results of data acquisition with the 22-lead ECG are less immediate than with standard 12-lead ECGs (18).

Efforts to improve the sensitivity and specificity for the detection of AMI and ischemia have included 15-lead ECG (a standard 12-lead ECG with the additional leads V_{4R}, V_8, and V_9) (3) and 22-lead ECG (a standard 12-lead ECG with additional unipolar leads distributed at specific locations on the anterior and posterior thorax) (18).

CRITIQUE
Scientific Basis

Right Ventricular Leads: A plethora of articles have assessed the diagnostic value of V_{4R} and other right-sided leads to detect RVI. There is a consensus that within this context, right-sided leads detect RVI with a sensitivity of 80% to 90% and a specificity of 80%. Most recently, Zehender and colleagues' work (7) showed that right ventricular leads are independent predictors of in-hospital and longterm prognosis in inferior-wall AMI.

Posterior Leads: Posterior-wall AMI usually occurs in the setting of inferior AMI but occurs as an isolated phenomenon about 5% of the time. Posterior leads occasionally have been reported to assist in the diagnosis of AMI. However, detecting "true" posterior-wall AMI from the numerous noninfarct cases is difficult, partly because it is an uncommon finding. Although the literature has documented that the standard 12-lead ECG is insensitive for detecting posterior AMI, there have been only occasional reports comparing findings on the standard 12-lead with those of posterior leads.

Body-Surface Mapping and Chaos Analysis: There is a fairly extensive collection of literature on body-surface mapping that shows its improved sensitivity and specificity compared with the standard 12-lead ECG in the diagnosis of AMI. However, the complexity of interpretation of body-surface leads appears to outweigh any advantage in accuracy or sensitivity. Chaos analysis is the subject of only one report (18), and its methods have not been examined by others.

Clinical Practicality

The complexity of the technology and interpretation limits the clinical application of body-surface mapping in a broad range of chest pain patients. For body-surface mapping, questions arise regarding its practicality and diffusability. There are no trials to address these concerns. Body-surface mapping appears to still be in the experimental and exploratory stage of development. There are no widely accepted, standardized lead systems that are easy to apply. Physicians need to be trained to interpret the new printouts in some of the developing systems. Clinical practicality has not been evaluated. Body-surface mapping studies are usually performed in the CCU, and this technology has not been tested as an ED-based technology.

Right-sided leads are placed as easily and conveniently as conventional leads. Posterior leads are sometimes inconvenient to place; however, flat strip leads have replaced suction cups, making administration much easier. The nonstandard ECG leads are direct extensions of the standard 12 leads, which minimizes interpretation difficulties. The 22-lead ECG is a technology unfamiliar to most practicing clinicians.

Data from Prospective Trials in the ED Setting

Studies of Test Sensitivity and Specificity: Zalenski et al (3) applied 15-lead ECGs in an ED setting to 149 patients admitted with suspected AMI (V_8, V_9, V_{4R}) or unstable angina. Major abnormalities (ST-segment deviation, T-wave inversion, Q waves) were found on the extra three leads in 28.9% of patients (43 of 149). Sensitivity of ST-segment elevation for AMI on 12 versus 15 leads increased from 47.1% (16 of 34) to 58.8% (20 of 34), respectively, with no decrease in specificity. McNemar's pair-matched analysis for ST-segment elevation on an AMI subgroup showed an association of ST elevation with the 15-lead ECG ($P < 0.05$) (3). Analysis of ECG criteria for thrombolytic therapy presenting uniquely on extra leads showed an increased sensitivity from 35.3% (12 of 34) to 44.1% (15 of 34) on 12 versus 15 leads, respectively; 13.5% of patients who did not meet criteria on 12 leads did so on 15 leads. The authors concluded that the 15-lead ECG provided increased sensitivity detecting ST-segment elevation in AMI patients with no loss of specificity. Its use may expand the selection of thrombolytic therapy candidates and provide a fuller ECG description of the extent of myocardial injury and necrosis. However, this sample was nonconsecutive, and ECGs were read by a cardiologist (blinded to outcomes); similar results may not be seen with readers not trained in cardiology.

Justis et al (18) applied a 22-lead ECG in an ED setting to 163 patients admitted with a cardiac-related diagnosis. Emergency physicians were blinded to the 22-lead ECG test results, and potential impact was retrospectively determined. The 22-lead ECG is designed to estimate deviations in myocardial conduction velocity that may be associated with clinically significant coronary artery disease. Data are acquired and analyzed in two equal sampling periods, summed over all 22 leads, and converted into an ischemic index ranging arbitrarily from 0 to 150. The 22-lead ECG provided a statistically significant improvement in sensitivity (83%) for AMI diagnosis over the 12-lead ECG (51%) with specificities of 76% and 99%, respectively. The authors concluded that when combined with clinical judgment, the 22-lead ECG could provide a 97.6% sensitivity for AMI diagnosis while reducing unnecessary admissions for AMI rule-out by 69%. This study has not been validated for the diagnosis of AMI and appears to be in an early developmental stage. In addition, it was actually less sensitive (73.7% versus 84%) for the AMI subgroup who received thrombolytic therapy. It may be that chaos analysis cannot distinguish epicardial injury patterns from other disturbed conduction signals produced by subendocardial ischemia.

Studies of the Clinical Impact of the Tests' Actual Use: None is reported.

Data from Other Clinical Settings

Posterior Leads: Melendez et al (19) studied the value of posterior leads in the detection of acute injury patterns. They reported posterior lead findings in 117 patients admitted to a monitored unit for suspected AMI. Three of 46 confirmed AMI patients (6.5%) demonstrated ST-segment elevation or Q waves solely on the posterior leads. Rich et al (2) reported that a Q wave of at least 40 milliseconds in V_9 was more specific and sensitive in the diagnosis of posterior wall AMI than standard criteria such as an R wave-to-S wave ratio of >1 in V_2.

Toyama et al (14) evaluated posterior leads V_7 to V_9 in the context of body-surface mapping. When body-surface mapping was used as diagnostic of posterior-wall AMI in the retrospective cohort, the addition of posterior leads increased the proportion of diagnostic ECGs from 5 of 20 to 11 of 20. Ikeda et al (16) showed that V_1 (R/S $>$ 1) is afflicted with a high false-negative rate in detection of old posterior infarction. Perloff (4) found the sensitivity of posterior leads for posterior-wall AMI (defined by vector-cardiogram criteria) in 10 patients to be 90%. However, Boden et al (20) found that anterior ST-segment depression (a common criterion for posterior reciprocal injury pattern) was only 46% predictive of posterior wall AMI. These studies suggest that leads V_8 and V_9 may be superior in the diagnosis of posterior-wall AMI to the reciprocal findings in leads V_1 to V_3. However, a definitive study comparing ECG and anatomic data is lacking.

Right Ventricular Infarction: Inferior AMI frequently involves the right ventricle. The presence of ST-segment elevation in lead V_{4R} in one study (7) was highly predictive of RVI (sensitivity, 88%; specificity, 78%; diagnostic accuracy, 83%) compared with other diagnostic procedures. Patients with ST-segment elevation in lead V_{4R} had a higher in-hospital mortality rate (31% versus 6%, $P <$ 0.001) and a higher incidence of major in-hospital complications (64% versus 28%, $P <$ 0.001) than did those without ST-segment elevation in lead V_{4R}. Multiple logistic-regression analysis showed ST-segment elevation in V_{4R} to be independent of and superior to all other clinical variables available on admission for the prediction of in-hospital mortality and major complications.

The authors of this study (7) concluded that right ventricular involvement during inferior AMI can be accurately diagnosed by the presence of ST-segment elevation in lead V_{4R}, a finding that is a strong, independent predictor of major complications and in-hospital mortality. ECG assessment or RVI should be performed routinely in all patients with inferior AMI.

In 1974, Erhardt (21) reported that CR_{4R}, a lead placed in the fifth intercostal space at the level of the right midclavicular line, showed ST-segment elevation of 1 mm or more in 10 of 17 patients with autopsy-documented RVI. A subsequent study demonstrated that ST-segment elevation in lead CR_{4R} was found to be 70% sensitive and 100% specific for the diagnosis of RVI and indicated right ventricular myocardial damage exceeding 25% or reaching the lateral margin of the right ventricular free wall (22). Candell–Riera et al (9) found that 52% of patients with inferior transmural AMI had ST-segment elevation in lead V_{4R}. Braat et al (8) found that ST-segment elevation of 1 mm or more in leads V_{3R}, V_{5R}, and V_{6R} was a reliable sign of RVI. V_{4R} was the lead with the greatest combined diagnostic sensitivity (93%) and predictive accuracy (93%). Croft et al (23) concluded that ST-segment elevation in one or more leads of V_{4R} to V_{5R} was highly sensitive (90%) and specific (91%) in identifying RVI and better than V_{4R} alone. Further investigations have confirmed the value of ST-segment elevation in lead V_{4R}, and in other right chest leads, for the detection of right ventricular AMI (10,11,24,25). V_{4R} is the lead that has more consistently shown a very high diagnostic sensitivity, specificity, and predictive accuracy.

Body-Surface Mapping: Ackaoui et al (26) found that there was a close relationship between body-surface mapping and abnormal segmental left ventricular wall motion and that body-surface mapping was "slightly" better than ECG for the diagnosis of AMI. Walker et al (27) suggested that the considerations of maximal ST-segment elevation and maximal ST-segment depression and their differences can predict poor prognosis subsets of an inferior AMI. Their study also shows that electrode malposition can affect the standard 12-lead assessment of ST-segment displacements (27). Another study applying 87 unipolar ECG leads distributed over the entire thoracic surface demonstrated that body-surface mapping is a sensitive and specific method to detect posterior-wall infarction (16).

Kornreich et al (28) compared 120-lead body-surface mapping

data from 131 AMI patients and 159 normal control subjects. The leads were assessed by having patients wear a vest that required only 5 minutes from approaching the ECG to obtaining the tracing. Sensitivity was 95% for AMI compared with 88% for 12-lead ECG. The use of body-surface mapping identified areas on the torso where the most significant ST-segment changes occur most frequently. Five of the six leads that were found to yield maximal detection of AMI and discrimination from normal findings were outside the standard precordial positions. The authors concluded that appropriate selection of ECG leads may help remove inconsistencies in current ECG diagnosis. However, it may be problematic checking bad chest leads and correcting baseline drift. Also, their results were not reproduced prospectively on a large representative sample, and no valid program is available to interpret large lead systems.

Like vectorcardiography, body-surface mapping is a research tool to be used in investigational settings. Its principal role appears to be to further define the applications and limitations of the standard ECG.

Generalizability to Different Settings

Although no study of body-surface mapping has been done in the ED, the greatest potential value of such technologies is their application in the initial evaluation of chest pain patients to increase the sensitivity and specificity of the detection of ischemic syndromes. Extra-lead ECG monitoring in a CCU setting to assess the impact of interventional strategies and sensitively detect coronary artery reocclusion has not been studied. Application in the prehospital setting would have to demonstrate clinical practicality and alterations in patient care and outcome.

Applicability to Different Population Subgroups, Including Women and Minorities

Extra-lead ECG techniques can be applied to different population subgroups, including women and minorities. However, there are no data on differential sensitivity or specificity in women or minority patients.

Cost Considerations

No data were found on the cost of these technologies. However, common sense suggests that the marginal cost of adding one to six leads would be modest. Detection of RVI with lead V_{4R} and more sensitive and specific detection of posterior infarction with leads V_8 and V_9 are acquired with the universally available 12-lead electrocardiograph and, aside from three additional electrodes per ECG, require no additional capital expenditure. The 22-lead ECG and body-surface mapping techniques require a significant investment in additional technology costs and interpretation.

Special Concerns

The sensitivity and specificity of a test define only partially its inherent accuracy because accuracy is also dependent on the prevalence of disease in the population to which the test is applied. All extra-lead and body-surface mapping studies have been applied to carefully selected ischemic populations already determined to require hospital admission. Therefore the published accuracies do not apply to a broad range of chest pain patients who are either discharged from the ED or admitted to the hospital without a diagnosis of acute ischemic heart disease. Inclusion of discharged patients would alter determinations of sensitivity and specificity.

Extra-lead ECG complexes require educated and careful interpretation. Posterior leads frequently have low amplitude QRS complexes (<10 mm), and ST-segment elevation can be subtle and require careful interpretation. Widespread application of extra-lead ECG could result in interpretive error.

The use of lead V_{4R} to detect RVI should be applied early in the course of AMI because ST-segment elevation in V_{4R} is a transient phenomenon disappearing within 10 to 18 hours of chest pain onset.

Primary Advantages

Right Ventricular Leads: First, right ventricular leads directly assess areas that are inadequately assessed by the standard 12 leads. V_1 and V_2 do not reflect right ventricular activity. ECG tracings from right-sided leads are easy to acquire and are interpreted in the same way as conventional 12-lead ECGs. Multiple studies have replicated the findings regarding prognostic and management data. Recording these leads may alter risk-benefit ratios for thrombolytic therapy administration.

Posterior Leads: Posterior leads directly assess activity of the posterior wall. Findings of posterior-wall AMI on standard 12-lead are insensitive and not specific; even when findings are present on a

12-lead ECG, the diagnosis is frequently missed because of difficulty in detecting prominent R waves and in distinguishing anterior ischemia from posterior injury. Posterior leads may identify new thrombolytic or emergent angioplasty candidates and may increase sensitivity of AMI detection. Finally, associations of inferior and posterior injury patterns may provide an improved severity classification of infarctions and help refine the process of risk-benefit assessment for emergency interventions.

Chaos analysis The 22-lead ECG is a predictive instrument representing a significant investment in technology cost that requires further prospective validation in an ED setting to determine its clinical practicality and benefit. However, 22-lead ECGs have the potential to reduce unnecessary AMI rule-out admissions.

Body-Surface Mapping: Body-surface mapping, when retrospectively applied to selected ischemic patients, produces semiquantitative data regarding infarct size and location and is a more sensitive and specific method for the detection of posterior infarction than either the 12-lead ECG or the vectorcardiogram. Body-surface mapping appears to offer promise for increasing the sensitivity and specificity of resting ECG technology.

Primary Disadvantages

Right ventricular leads are not known to increase the sensitivity for AMI diagnosis or for identifying thrombolytic candidates; they are valuable primarily for management and prognosis.

Posterior leads have marginal utility as a result of the limited number of isolated true posterior AMIs. Also, there is limited knowledge regarding their sensitivity.

All extra-lead ECG and body-surface mapping studies have been performed only in select ischemic populations; therefore the estimates of sensitivity and specificity do not apply to larger chest pain populations who are either discharged or admitted to the hospital without a diagnosis of acute ischemic heart disease. Extra-lead ECGs require educated and careful evaluation to avoid interpretive error. There has not been a clinical effectiveness study that has demonstrated what improvements in diagnostic performance will be attained when nonstandard ECG leads are utilized in the course of routine care.

From the perspective of the Working Group, body-surface mapping has not been tested in the ED setting, and lead placement might delay patient care in receiving thrombolytic therapy.

Although efficacy trials suggest modest benefit, there are no validation or effectiveness trials. Finally, chaos analysis had a decreased sensitivity for the thrombolytic group.

SUMMARY AND RECOMMENDATIONS

Sampling right ventricular leads is clinically practical, uses the universally available 12-lead ECG, and appears to increase the sensitivity and specificity for detection of RVI (a strong, independent predictor of major complications and in-hospital mortality in patients with inferior AMI). Such leads have the potential to improve severity classification of AMIs, help refine the process of risk-benefit assessment for emergency interventions, possibly provide an indication for thrombolytic treatment, and avoid nitrate-induced hypotension in patients with RVI. Sampling posterior leads may also improve the sensitivity of the ECG for posterior AMI. Larger prospective studies applied in a variety of EDs with a broader range of admitted and discharged chest pain patients are required to determine the risks and benefits of this technology. If sensitivity and specificity are comparable to the standard 12-lead ECG, then studies to assess clinical impact in the ED would be warranted.

The 22-lead ECG is a predictive instrument that requires prospective ED evaluation and a cost analysis to assess its clinical practicality and benefit.

Body-surface mapping is a valuable research tool requiring specialized equipment for acquisition and specialized software for processing the information. This is not currently practical for ED patient assessment. However, the improved sensitivity and specificity suggested by preliminary efficacy type trials indicate that this approach may eventually contribute to the ED diagnosis of acute cardiac ischemia.

Table 5-1   Nonstandard ECG Leads and Body-Surface Mapping

	ED Diagnostic Performance		ED Clinical Impact	
	Quality of Evidence	Accuracy	Quality of Evidence	Impact
Nonstandard ECG leads	C	+	NK	NK
Body-surface mapping	NK	NK	NK	NK

The results of the Working Group's final ratings of the quality of evidence evaluating these technologies and of their ED diagnostic performance and clinical impact are detailed in Table 5-1.

REFERENCES

1. Rude RE, Poole WK, Muller JE, et al. Electrocardiographic and clinical criteria for recognition of acute myocardial infarction based on analysis of 3,697 patients. *Am J Cardiol* 1983; 52:936–942.

2. Rich MW, Imburgia M, King TR, et al. Electrocardiographic diagnosis of remote posterior wall myocardial infarction using unipolar posterior lead V_9. *Chest* 1989;96:489–493.

3. Zalenski RJ, Cooke D, Rydman R, et al. Assessing the diagnostic value of an ECG containing leads V_{4R}, V_8, and V_9: the 15-lead ECG. *Ann Emerg Med* 1993;22:786–793.

4. Perloff JK. The recognition of strictly posterior myocardial infarction by conventional scale electrocardiography. *Circulation* 1964;30:706–718.

5. Seyal MS, Swiryn S. True posterior myocardial infarction. *Arch Intern Med* 1983;143:983–985.

6. Dunn RF, Newman HN, Vemstein L. The clinical features of isolated left circumflex coronary artery disease. *Circulation* 1984;69(3):477–484.

7. Zehender M, Kasper W, Kauder E, et al. Right ventricular infarction as an independent predictor of prognosis after acute inferior myocardial infarction. *N Engl J Med* 1993;328(14):981–988.

8. Braat SH, Bruguda P, den Dulk K, et al. Value of lead V_{4R} for recognition of the infarct coronary artery in acute myocardial infarction. *Am J Cardiol* 1984;53:1538–1541.

9. Candell-Riera J, Figueras J, Vaile V, et al. Right ventricular infarction: relationships between ST segment elevation in V_{4R} and hemodynamic, scintigraphic, and echocardiographic findings in patients with acute inferior myocardial infarction. *Am Heart J* 1981;101:281–287.

10. Klein HO, Tordiman T, Ninio R, et al. The early recognition of right ventricular infarction. Diagnostic accuracy of the electrocardiographic V_{4R} lead. *Circulation* 1983;67:558–565.

11. Lopez-Sendon J, Coma-Canella I, Alcasena S, et al. Electrocardiographic findings in acute right ventricular infarction: sensitivity and specificity of electrocardiographic alterations of right

precordial leads V_{4R}, V_{3R}, V_1, V_2, and V_3. *J Am Coll Cardiol* 1985; 19(6):1273–1279.

12. Maroko PR, Libby P, Govell JW, et al. Precordial ST segment elevation mapping: an atraumatic method for assessing alterations in the extent of myocardial ischemic injury. *Am J Cardiol* 1972;29:223–230.

13. Madias JE. A comparison of serial 49-lead precordial ECG maps and standard 6-lead precordial ECGs in patients with acute anterior Q wave myocardial infarction. *J Electrocardiol* 1989;22:113–124.

14. Toyama S, Suzuki K, Yoshino K, et al. A comparative study of body surface isopotential mapping and the electrocardiogram in diagnosing myocardial infarction. *J Electrocardiol* 1984;17: 7–13.

15. Gobel F, Tschida VH. Screening yield of electrocardiogram chaos analysis in low-risk individuals. *Circulation* 1990;82(suppl III):III–619.

16. Ikeda K, Kubota I, Tonooka I, et al. Detection of posterior myocardial infarction by body surface mapping: a comparative study with 12 lead ECG and VCG. *J Electrocardiol* 1985;18: 361–369.

17. Braunwald E, Maroko PR. ST-segment mapping: realistic and unrealistic expectations (editorial). *Circulation* 1976;54:529–532.

18. Justis DL, Hession WT. Accuracy of 22-lead ECG analysis for diagnosis of acute myocardial infarction and coronary artery disease in the emergency department: a comparison with 12-lead ECG. *Ann Emerg Med* 1992;21:1–9.

19. Melendez LJ, Jones DT, Salcedo JR. Usefulness of three additional electrocardiographic chest leads (V_7, V_8, and V_9) in the diagnosis of acute myocardial infarction. *Can Med Assoc J* 1978; 119:745–748.

20. Boden WE, Kleiger RE, Gibson RS, et al. Electrocardiographic evolution of posterior acute myocardial infarction: importance of early precordial ST-segment depression. *Am J Cardiol* 1987; 59:782–787.

21. Erhardt LR. Clinical and pathological observations in different types of acute myocardial infarction: a study of 84 patients deceased after treatment in a coronary care unit. *Acta Med Scand* 1974;26(suppl 560):7–78.

22. Erhardt LR, Sjogren A, Wahiberg I. Single right-sided precordial lead in the diagnosis of right ventricular involvement

in inferior myocardial infarction. *Am Heart J* 1976;91:571–576.

23. Croft CH, Nicod P, Corbett JR. Detection of acute right ventricular infarction by right precordial electrocardiography. *Am J Cardiol* 1982;50:421–427.

24. Morgera T, Albert E, Silvestri F, et al. Right precordial ST and QRS changes in the diagnosis of right ventricular infarction. *Am Heart J* 1984;108:13–18.

25. Lew AS, Laramee P, Shah PK, et al. Ratio of ST-segment depression in lead V_2 to ST-segment elevation in lead V_2 to ST-segment elevation in lead aVF in evolving inferior acute myocardial infarction: an aid to the early recognition of right ventricular ischemia. *Am J Cardiol* 1986;57:1047–1051.

26. Ackaoui A, Nadeau R, Sestier F, et al. Myocardial infarction diagnosis with body surface potential mapping, electrocardiography, vectorcardiography and thallium-201 scintigraphy: a correlative study with left ventriculography. *Clin Invest Med* 1985;8(1):68–77.

27. Walker SJ, Bell AJ, Loughhead MG, et al. Spatial distribution and prognostic significance of ST segment potential determined by body surface mapping in patients with acute inferior AMI. *Circulation* 1987;76(2):289–297.

28. Kornreich F, Rautaharlu PM, Warren J, et al. Identification of best electrocardiographic leads for diagnosing myocardial infarction by statistical analysis of body surface potential maps. *Am J Cardiol* 1985;56:852–856.

ECG Exercise Stress Test

6

SUMMARY OF TECHNOLOGY

The ECG exercise stress test would be used in selected subgroups after AMI and recurrent rest ischemic syndromes have been ruled out in the initial workup. It would not be used for general or early detection. The purpose of an ED ECG stress test would be to evaluate the patient for exercise-induced ischemia and determine prognosis for cardiac events. A negative test result may allow the patient to be discharged from the ED and worked up further as an outpatient. Given the ease with which an ECG stress test may be performed, there is interest in the utility of the test in a population of low- to moderate-risk patients, in whom the triage decision is not clear.

Multiple treadmill protocols are in use (1,2), including the Bruce protocol and others such as the Naughton, Weber, and Balke Ware, which are more appropriate for patients with limited exercise tolerance. Lead placement is per the Mason-Likar modification of the standard 12-lead ECG, which moves limb leads toward the chest and hips. ECGs are taken at baseline, at the end of each stage, with any symptoms, immediately before and after stopping exercise, and for each minute of recovery until heart rate or ECGs return to baseline. Blood pressure is monitored frequently, and continuous telemetry is performed. An exercise technician and a physician generally perform the test. Nearby resuscitative equipment is mandatory (3). Contraindications to a routine ECG stress test include known unstable angina with recent chest pain, uncompensated heart failure, untreated arrhythmias, critical aortic stenosis, myocarditis/pericarditis, and uncontrolled hypertension. These diagnoses would necessarily need to be excluded by the emergency medicine physician.

ST-segment depression is the hallmark of ischemia and can be horizontal, upsloping, or downsloping, with different degrees of positivity. Ischemia is diagnosed by: 1) 1.5 mm upsloping ST-segment depression 60 to 80 milliseconds beyond the J point or 2) 1.0 mm horizontal to downsloping ST-segment depression at the J point, beyond the isoelectric point (TP segment) in three consecutive ECG complexes. ST-segment elevation is also considered ischemic when not located in an area of prior infarct. T-wave changes are not sensitive for ischemia. Computer analyses are available to assist with interpretation but cannot be relied on solely.

The use of bayesian theory incorporates the pretest likelihood, based on patient risk, sensitivity, and specificity of the test, to calculate the posttest probability given the clinical results. Risk is determined by the history of chest pain, risk factors, age, and sex of the patient. The clinical results include the extent of ST-segment depression noted at maximal work capacity. Patterson and Horowitz (4) demonstrated that optimal posttest probability is found in patients with an intermediate pretest likelihood of coronary disease.

CRITIQUE
Scientific Basis

Only low-risk patients have been subjected to ECG stress testing in the ED, and the test is recognized to be of lower yield in any low-risk population. The value of exercising patients in the ED is to reduce unnecessary admissions and to complete what is otherwise a routine outpatient diagnostic test.

The gold standard for determining accuracy of an ECG stress test has been coronary angiography, with a 50% to 70% coronary artery stenosis as the definition of a significant lesion. Length of lesion, serial lesions, and coronary vascular reserve have not been taken into account in these studies, and the reference standard is not ideal. The sensitivity and specificity of the single criterion of 1 mm ST-segment depression are 50% to 70% for single vessel disease and 80% to 90% for three-vessel disease (5). Pfisterer et al (6) found a 58% sensitivity and 71% specificity. In a population with a high prevalence of atypical chest pain, Goodin et al (7) found a specificity of 64%. Logistic regression shows that a positive ST-segment response raises the posttest probability to 20% to 40% even for patients with very low pretest probabilities (8). Referral bias in all studies decreases the rate of true-negative tests and increases the rate of false-positive tests, thus increasing sensitivity and decreasing specificity.

A problem with estimating the usefulness of ECG exercise stress testing arises because there is a consensus that its sensitivity and specificity are not independent of the tested population. Factors that affect sensitivity include maximal heart rate achieved, number of diseased vessels, type of angina, age, and sex (9). Sensitivity and specificity data are always developed from patients who ultimately get cardiac catheterization, which may reflect a posttest referral bias. Because this often does not represent the population to whom it is applied, the yield estimates made using the reported diagnostic values may be inaccurate.

A patient to whom an ED-based ECG stress test is administered would likely have pretest probabilities of coronary artery disease (CAD) between 10% and 25%. Interpretation of the test would be based on the development of symptoms and electrocardiographic changes, considering the patient's prior probability of CAD. When using a cutoff of 1 mm or greater ST-segment depression, the sensitivity and specificity of an ECG stress test are approximately 68% and 77%, respectively (10). If in a low-prevalence population the sensitivity for CAD is assumed to be modestly worse than that (eg, 60%) and the specificity better (eg, 90%), then a pretest probability of 10% would have a posttest probability of 40% if positive and 5% if negative. If the pretest probability were 20%, the posttest results would be 60% and 10%, respectively. Because the sensitivity for detecting three-vessel disease is higher, the posttest probability will be higher for detecting this condition. Thus ECG stress testing could partition pretest probability patients of 10% to 20% into a higher probability group (40% to 60%) and a lower probability group (5% to 10%).

Clinical Practicality

Outpatient emergency ECG exercise stress testing has been performed in several situations. Patients can be held over in the ED/observation unit until the services are available in the hospital. Alternatively, chest pain units have been set up to provide ECG stress testing for ED patients with chest pain (11). Cardiologists have traditionally overseen and interpreted ECG exercise stress testing in hospitals, and there would be the need to train other physicians or provide immediate interpretation for these services.

There will be a significant population of patients who will not be eligible for standard exercise treadmill stress testing as a result of abnormalities of the baseline ECG (ECG with left ventricular hypertrophy (LVH), left bundle-branch block, or patient on digoxin) or to very poor exercise reserve.

Reasonable eligibility criteria for an early ECG stress test would be necessary before widespread use in the ED. The group to be targeted are patients at moderate probability of having CAD—in other words, patients in whom the suspicion of CAD is high enough to consider admission to the hospital but low enough so that the decision is questionable (12).

Data from Prospective Clinical Trials in the ED Setting

Studies of Test Sensitivity and Specificity: Studies of test sensitivity and specificity have not been performed specifically for the ED setting. The Working Group considers that the same general limitations of ECG exercise stress testing found in the outpatient setting will apply to the ED.

Studies of the Clinical Impact of the Test's Actual Use: In a large sample of patients evaluated in a chest pain center located in the ED, 791 of 1,010 patients underwent graded ECG exercise stress testing after 9 hours of nondiagnostic serial ECG/ST-segment trend monitoring; 0-, 3-, 6-, and 9-hour CK-MB testing; and resting echocardiography (11). None of the patients undergoing ECG exercise stress testing sustained an adverse event while being tested. Of these 791 patients, 782 (98.9%) had negative or nondiagnostic ECG stress tests, and the positive predictive value was 44% (four of nine) for CAD. Thirty-day follow-up revealed a 0.1% AMI rate and 0.5% all-cause mortality rate; four of five deaths were noncardiac, and one was of unknown cause. Kerns et al (13) prospectively studied 32 young patients (women ages 18 to 49 years, men ages 18 to 39 years) with atypical chest pain, normal ECGs, and 0-to-1 risk factor for CAD from 1990 to 1991 to evaluate the feasibility, safety, and reliability of this method. They compared these results with those of a retrospective sample of similar patients who were admitted. Any patient with a moderate suspicion of AMI or ischemic heart disease, two or more cardiac risk factors, prior documentation of CAD, history of insulin or non–insulin-dependent diabetes mellitus, use of β- or calcium-channel blockers or digoxin, prior hypertension treatment or ED blood pressure greater than 160/95 mm Hg, cocaine use, inability to use the treadmill, or presentations when treadmill testing was not available were excluded from the study. All tests were interpreted as normal without clinical events for 6-month follow-up. The control group likewise had normal ECG stress test results, but the average length of stay was 2 days, at a cost of $2,340. The cost of the expedited workup was $467 for an average stay of 5.5 hours.

Kerns and colleagues (13) appropriately reviewed the limitations of their study: The low-risk patient population had a pretest likelihood of 20%, which was reduced to less than 10% after an ECG stress test. Only normal ECGs were included, already a low-risk population, because of the difficulties of standard ECG interpretation with baseline repolarization abnormalities. Patients with potentially blunted maximal heart rates (as a result of medications) were also excluded. Sample bias may have been introduced because only daytime ECG stress tests were performed, eliminating the patient population with nocturnal rest symptoms. Studies of higher-risk patients are clearly indicated.

Tsakonis et al (14) also reviewed the safety of immediate treadmill testing in selected ED patients with chest pain, again using small numbers (28 patients) of low-risk patients (normal ECGs). They performed an early ECG exercise stress test (within several hours) but admitted all patients despite negative test results. Follow-up at 6 months again was negative. They suggested that a negative ECG stress test in the ED could preclude unnecessary hospitalizations.

Zalenski et al (15) studied patients with chest pain and suspected AMI or ACI who needed admission and were low risk for AMI according to the protocol developed by Goldman et al (16). Patients were excluded if they had clinical angina, were hemodynamically unstable, and had baseline ECG abnormalities or clinical parameters (such as severe anemia or hypertension) that precluded an ECG stress test. Of 96 patients assigned to the protocol workup, 2% were classified as having AMI, 12.6% as having unstable angina, 9.5% as being no longer eligible or other diagnosis, and 75.8% as having no ischemia. Of the group that had ECG stress tests, 67% were conclusively negative, 9.1% were positive, and 24.2% were inconclusive. Patient acceptance of the ECG stress test at any hour of the day was high. Outcomes on sensitivity and specificity of ECG exercise stress testing await publication.

Data from Other Clinical Studies

Gianrossi et al (17) performed a metaanalysis of 147 published studies involving 24,074 patients who underwent both ECG exercise stress testing and coronary angiography. The mean sensitivity was 68% (range, 23% to 100%), and the mean specificity was 77% (range, 17% to 100%). Detrano et al (5) reported that patients with three-vessel disease had a higher sensitivity (81%; range, 40% to 100%) and lower specificity (66%; range, 17% to 100%). The weighted mean sensitivity was 86% ± 11%, and mean specificity was 53% ± 24% for left main or three-vessel disease.

There is extensive literature on diagnostic ECG exercise stress testing in different patient populations. Prognostic as well as diagnostic data are available (18–21). Mark et al (18) developed a treadmill score that added independent prognostic information to clinical data already available, including coronary anatomy and left ventricular ejection fraction. The score incorporated exercise time, ST deviation, and angina to identify patients at high versus low risk for 5-year mortality. Studies by Fruergaard et al (19) and Madsen et al (20) of patients in whom AMI was ruled out are useful to examine. These researchers found that patients in whom AMI was ruled out, who had no other cardiac diagnosis, and who had exercise—but not resting—ST-segment depression, had a 10% higher rate of cardiac events (87.8% versus 97.6%) after 12 months of follow-up (1% per month).

Lewis and Amsterdam (22) presented preliminary data on the comparative utility of "immediate" ECG exercise stress testing on men and women. All patients were admitted with a chest pain syndrome and underwent ECG exercise stress testing within 24 hours, before enzymes were completely available. They had a positive rate of 12% (12% men, 13% women), 8 of 10 of whom had additional testing. There were three true-positive tests (two men, one woman) and five false positives (two men, three women). The positive predictive value was 38%. There was no difference in 6-month follow-up in either men or women who had negative or nondiagnostic test results. The authors concluded that there is no sex bias in patient selection for an immediate ECG stress test, but this study was not in an ED setting.

The safety of ECG exercise stress testing in the non-selected patient population has been demonstrated, with mortality rates of less than 0.01% and morbidity of less than 0.05% (23). Risks increase if a patient is tested within 4 weeks of an infarct and are doubled when a symptom-limited (maximal) rather than a low-level protocol is used.

Generalizability to Different Settings

Current ED studies are very limited, and therefore the results cannot be generalized. Although conclusions from inpatient studies are probably close to those for the ED chest paint patient population, important differences may be present due to the more acute nature of the latter. Additional data on the prognostic and diagnostic value of the ECG stress test for ED patients need to be collected.

Applicability to Population Subgroups, Including Women and Minorities

Standard exercise literature is replete with studies demonstrating decreased specificity of exercise-induced ST-segment changes in women, in part as a result of a lower prevalence and extent of CAD in premenopausal women (24). Some studies have found different prognostic values of ECG stress test results for women (25). Therefore it will be important to consider the patients' prior probability of CAD when administering an ECG stress test. More recent work focuses on the underevaluation and treatment of women with CAD.

Patients with hypertension, more prevalent in blacks than in other ethnic groups, may experience less benefit from ECG exercise stress testing because of difficulty in interpretation if baseline repolarization changes from LVH are present. Exclusion due to the presence of LVH may be a greater problem in the black population given the higher prevalence of hypertension. Further studies would be necessary to look at this population specifically.

Cost Considerations

There would be modest costs to set up and staff a stress laboratory off the ED. There would be space requirements, treadmill costs, and at least one full-time employee who is certified in Basic Life Support/Advanced Cardiac Life Support. Traditionally, the tests are performed with a physician in the immediate vicinity, but with this higher-risk patient, theoretically the physician would be supervising tests directly. The hours of operation would be dictated by the frequency and volume of testing.

Alternatively, the current stress laboratories could be utilized if an observation unit is available that could hold patients for less than 24 hours. Again, the impact of these "immediate" tests may decompress some of the scheduled inpatient as well as outpatient examinations. At a potential $1,873 savings per test, there could be a significant reduction of unnecessary admissions. However, if only very low risk patients receive an ECG exercise stress test, the savings may be less due to false-positive findings.

Special Concerns

It may be very difficult to determine a set of criteria to identify patients at low-to-moderate risk of CAD in whom ECG exercise stress testing will be helpful in determining triage. Truly low-risk patients for CAD should not undergo a test that has little chance of significantly altering the posttest likelihood of ACI, which may lead to overtesting of nondiseased patients. Having this technology available may generate overutilization of ECG exercise stress testing in the ED. Positive results are likely to be false positives in a very low risk patient population. There are currently no prospective randomized trials to evaluate the utility of the ECG stress test in the ED.

New likelihood ratios would be helpful, because ED chest pain patients may have different acuity and severity from patients referred from office visits. Until a moderate-risk patient is able to undergo this testing safely, probably on a modified protocol, its practical utility is limited. The interpreted results must also be available immediately, which requires special skills, training, and the cooperation of emergency medicine, cardiology, and primary care staff.

In a national survey of ECG exercise stress testing, Stuart and Ellestad (23) reported 3.58 per 10,000 patient tests had AMI, 4.78 arrhythmias, and 0.5 deaths, for an overall complication rate of 8.86/10,000 tests. Malani et al (26) reported complications occurring in 1.8% (n = 1,000) composed of arrhythmias, hypotension, or angina, but no AMI or death. It remains to be seen whether ECG exercise stress testing immediately after a period of ED observation yields higher complication rates. Thus far, no complications have been reported in the reports of early ECG exercise stress testing (0 per 851; 95% CI, 0 to 0.4%).

Data on ECG exercise stress testing to date have been analyzed based on rigid cardiologist ECG interpretation of well-defined patient subsets (age, sex, classification of chest pain, ST-segment negativity, risk factor status, etc). There is a national trend toward generalists performing and interpreting their own exercise stress tests. Although not specifically related to ED issues, a report from Scotland (27) documented that different hospitals are inconsistent in patient selection, test conditions, and interpretation of ECG stress test results. In the United States, rigid standardization of ECG exercise stress-testing interpretation must be maintained, as has been put forth by the American Heart Association (3,28).

Primary Advantages

Completing an expeditious diagnostic workup may reduce the number of unnecessary admissions for chest pain. ECG exercise stress testing in the ED is an efficient and convenient procedure that is potentially cost saving and can provide immediate reassurance for the patient. An ECG stress test is a well-accepted testing method to evaluate a patient for significant CAD. It is relatively inexpensive and can be performed and interpreted by noncardiologists. The ready availability of resuscitation facilities in the ED helps address concerns over limited safety data.

Primary Disadvantages

Many groups of patients will be excluded from this method of testing as a result of uninterpretable baseline ECGs or poor exercise tolerance. There are no current randomized trials testing this methodology. Sensitivity, specificity, and safety have not been specifically determined for the ED acute chest pain population. ECG exercise stress testing is expected to add little if patients tested have moderate (>30%) or very low (<5%) pretest probability. The cost-effectiveness in the ED setting has not been determined. The acceptability to ED physicians has not been assessed; EDs may be too busy to devote space or personnel to this endeavor.

SUMMARY AND RECOMMENDATIONS

Currently there are limited data studying the impact of ECG exercise stress testing in the ED. Where the risk of CAD is low to moderate, the expedited ECG exercise stress test may offer the benefit of an expedited workup and may reduce hospital admissions for

Table 6-1   ECG Exercise Stress Test

ED Diagnostic Performance		ED Clinical Impact	
Quality of Evidence	Accuracy	Quality of Evidence	Impact
C	+	C	NK-NE

chest pain. Observation exercise status, where the patient is observed pending definitive testing, may offer a similar benefit. However, ECG exercise stress testing in the ED cannot be recommended in the absence of additional data demonstrating safety and effectiveness.

The results of the Working Group's final ratings of the quality of evidence evaluating this technology and of its ED diagnostic performance and clinical impact is set forth in Table 6-1.

REFERENCES

1. Froelicher VF, Marcondes GD. *Manual of Exercise Testing.* Chicago: Year Book, 1989.
2. Ellestad MH. *Stress Testing. Principles and Practice.* 3rd ed. Philadelphia: FA Davis, 1986.
3. Fletcher GF, Froelicher VF, Hartley LH, et al. Exercise standards. A statement for health professionals from the American Heart Association. *Circulation* 1990;82:2286–2322.
4. Patterson RE, Horowitz SF. Importance of epidemiology and biostatistics in deciding clinical strategies for using diagnostic tests: a simplified approach using examples from coronary artery disease. *J Am Coll Cardiol* 1989;13(7):1653–1665.
5. Detrano R, Gianrossi R, Mulvihill D, et al. Exercise-induced ST segment depression in the diagnosis of multivessel coronary artery disease: a meta analysis. *J Am Coll Cardiol* 1989;14(6):1501–1508.
6. Pfisterer ME, Williams RJ, Gordon DG, et al. Comparison of rest/exercise ECG, thallium-201 scans and radionuclide angiography in patients with unsuspected CAD. *Cardiology* 1980;66(1):43–55.
7. Goodin RR, Graham JM, Gwinn JS, et al. Exercise stress testing in patients with chest pain and normal coronary arteriography. *Cathet Cardiovasc Diagn* 1975;1(3):251–259.
8. Currie PJ, Kelly MJ, Harper RW, et al. Incremental value of clinical assessment, supine exercise ECG, and biplane exercise radionuclide ventriculography in the prediction of coronary artery disease in men with chest pain. *Am J Cardiol* 1983;52:927–935.
9. Hlatky MA, Pryor DB, Harrell F. Factors affecting sensitivity and specificity of exercise electrocardiography. *Am J Med* 1984;77:64–71.
10. Patterson RE, Eisner RL, Horowitz SF. Comparison of cost-

effectiveness and utility of exercise ECG, single photon emission computed tomography, positron emission tomography, and coronary angiography for the diagnosis of coronary artery disease. *Circulation* 1995;91:54–65.

11. Gibler WB, Runyon JP, Levy RC, et al. A rapid diagnostic treatment center for patients with chest pain in the emergency department. *Ann Emerg Med* 1995;25:1–8.

12. Gaspoz JM, Lee TH, Cook EF, et al. Outcome of patients who were admitted to a new short-stay unit to "rule-out" AMI. *Am J Cardiol* 1991;68:145–149.

13. Kerns JR, Shaub TF, Fontanarosa PB. Emergency cardiac stress testing in the evaluation of emergency department patients with atypical chest pain. *Ann Emerg Med* 1993;22:794–798.

14. Tsakonis JS, Shesser R, Rosenthal R, et al. Safety of immediate treadmill testing in selected emergency department patients with chest pain—a preliminary report. *Am J Emerg Med* 1991; 9:557–559.

15. Zalenski R, Roberts R, Das K, et al. Admission avoidance for chest pain patients (abstract). *Acad Emerg Med* 1994;1(2):A78.

16. Goldman L, Cook EF, Brand DA, et al. A computer protocol to predict myocardial infarction in emergency department patients with chest pain. *N Engl J Med* 1988;318:797–803.

17. Gianrossi R, Detrano R, Mulvihill D, et al. Exercise-induced ST depression in the diagnosis of coronary artery disease: a meta analysis. *Circulation* 1989;80(1):87–98.

18. Mark DB, Hlatky MA, Harrell FE, et al. Exercise treadmill score for predicting prognosis in coronary artery disease. *Ann Intern Med* 1987;106(6):793–800.

19. Fruergaard P, Launbjerg J, Jacobsen HL, et al. Seven-year prognostic value of the electrocardiogram at rest and an exercise test in patients admitted for, but without, confirmed myocardial infarction. *Eur Heart J* 1993;14:499–504.

20. Madsen JK, Hommel E, Hansen JF. Prognostic value of an electrocardiogram at rest and exercise test in patients admitted with suspected acute myocardial infarction, in whom the diagnosis is not confirmed. *Eur Heart J* 1987;8:717–724.

21. Bogaty P, Dagenais GR, Cantin B. Prognosis in patients with a strongly positive exercise electrocardiogram. *Am J Cardiol* 1989;64:1284–1288.

22. Lewis WR, Amsterdam EA. Comparative utility of immediate exercise testing in men and women presenting to the emer-

gency room with chest pain (abstract). *J Am Coll Cardiol* 1993; 21(2)(suppl A):238A.

23. Stuart RJ Jr, Ellestad MH. National survey of exercise stress testing facilities. *Chest* 1980;77:94–97.

24. Pratt CM, Francis MJ, Divine GW, et al. Exercise testing in women with chest pain. Are there additional exercise characteristics that predict true positive test results? *Chest* 1989;95(1): 139–144.

25. Manca C, Dei-Cas L, Albertinit D, et al. Different prognostic value of exercise electrocardiograph in men and women. *Cardiology* 1978;63(5):312–319.

26. Malani SK, Roy CP, Nath CS, et al. Complications in 1000 consecutive treadmill tests. *J Assoc Physicians India* 1993;4(8): 516–517.

27. Muir KW, Rodger JC, DeBono JS, et al. A survey of exercise testing practice in Scottish hospitals. *Scott Med J* 1993;38(2): 45–47.

28. American College of Cardiology/American Heart Association Task Force on Assessment of Cardiovascular Procedures (Subcommittee on Exercise Testing). Guidelines for exercise testing. *J Am Coll Cardiol* 1986;8(3):725–738.

Original ACI Predictive Instrument

7

SUMMARY OF TECHNOLOGY

Given that more than half of hospital admissions for presumed ACI prove to be falsely positive, an ideal diagnostic aid for ACI would increase physicians' diagnostic specificity without decreasing their already high diagnostic sensitivity. The purpose of the original Boston City Hospital Predictive Instrument Trial (1) and the Multicenter Predictive Instrument Trial (2) was to develop an easy-to-use method to improve emergency physicians' triage decisions so that fewer patients *without* ACI would be admitted to CCUs without decreasing the proper admission of patients *with* ACI. Reasoning that a single numerical probability value might be easily incorporated into physicians' clinical decisionmaking processes, the ACI predictive instrument trials sought to develop and prospectively test a mathematical instrument that could provide ED physicians with a patient's calculated likelihood of having ACI. The studies each had two 1-year phases: 1) development of the predictive instrument and 2) a prospective trial of its use in the participating hospitals' EDs (2).

The Boston City Hospital study (1) was the pilot for the Multicenter Predictive Instrument Trial (2), which sought to generalize the validity of the approach. Therefore the multicenter trial included a wide range of hospital types: two urban major teaching centers, two teaching-affiliate hospitals in smaller cities, and two nonteaching rural hospitals. Because the predictive instruments created in both studies and their impact in both studies were essentially the same, only the larger study is reported here.

In the multicenter study, the predictive instrument was developed on the basis of data on the 2,801 study subjects seen in the six participating hospitals' EDs from March 1979 through February 1980. Beginning with 59 clinical features available to ED physicians, including clinical presentation, history, physical findings, ECG, sociodemographic characteristics, and coronary disease risk factors, an equation was developed that used only seven variables and that was applicable to all six hospitals. This mathematically based instrument provides an estimate of a patient's likelihood of having true ACI expressed as a value between 0% and 100%. Once programmed into a hand-held calculator, the actual use of the instrument requires less than 20 seconds of computation time. Phase 2 was an 11-month prospective trial of the predictive instrument's impact that included 2,320 patients who were seen in the six hospitals' EDs: 1,288 during experimental periods and 1,032 during control periods. The use of the predictive instrument markedly improved physicians' diagnostic performance and admission practices, as detailed below.

On the basis of the more than 1.5 million patients with suspected ACI admitted to CCUs every year in this country, a nationwide reduction in admissions comparable to the 30% decrease for those *without ACI* as seen in the predictive instrument trials would reduce the number of CCU admissions by more than 250,000 each year. Thus, if widely used, the original predictive instrument for ACI would seem likely to have significant medical and financial benefits.

However, despite considerable attention given the study on its release and continued interest, the original ACI predictive instrument has not become widely used. Appreciation of the cumbersome nature of the programmable calculator version led to the attempt to improve the attractiveness of its use, including the creation of a table with the original ACI predictive instrument's probability to increase its ease of use (Table 7-1) and the incorporation of the ACI-TIPI (time-insensitive predictive instrument) (3) (described in a separate review in this report) into the electrocardiograph (4) (Figure 7-1).

Figure 7-1 ACI time-insensitive predictive instrument.

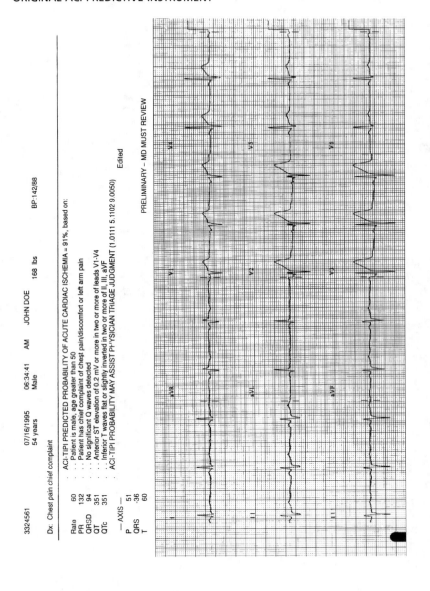

3324561   07/16/1995   06:34:41   AM   JOHN DOE   BP:142/88
                 54 years   Male   168 lbs

Dx: Chest pain chief complaint

Rate   60   ACI-TIPI PREDICTED PROBABILITY OF ACUTE CARDIAC ISCHEMIA = 91%, based on:
PR   132   . . Patient is male, age greater than 50
QRSD   94   . . Patient has chief complaint of chest pain/discomfort or left arm pain
QT   351   . . No significant Q waves detected
QTc   351   . . Anterior ST elevation of 0.2 mV or more in two or more of leads V1-V4
                . . Inferior T waves flat or slightly inverted in two or more of II, III, aVF
— AXIS —   . ACI-TIPI PROBABILITY MAY ASSIST PHYSICIAN TRIAGE JUDGMENT (1.0111 5.1102 9.0050)
P   51
QRS   -36   Edited
T   60

PRELIMINARY – MD MUST REVIEW

67

Table 7-1 The Original ACI Predictive Instrument's Probabilities of Acute Ischemia for ED Patients

Question: Chest pain or pressure, or left arm pain?
Answer: Yes, chief complaint.

	ECG Abnormalities (%)					
History	ST∅ T∅	ST— T∅	ST∅ T↑↓	ST↑↓ T∅	ST— T↑↓	ST↑↓ T↑↓
No heart attack *and* no NTG use	19	35	42	54	62	78
Either heart attack *or* NTG use (*not both*)	27	46	53	64	73	85
Both heart attack *and* NTG use	37	58	65	75	80	90

Answer: Yes, but not chief complaint.

	ECG Abnormalities (%)					
History	ST∅ T∅	ST— T∅	ST∅ T↑↓	ST↑↓ T∅	ST— T↑↓	ST↑↓ T↑↓
No heart attack *and* no NTG use	10	21	26	36	45	64
Either heart attack *or* NTG use (*not both*)	16	29	36	48	56	74
Both heart attack *and* NTG use	22	40	47	59	67	82

Answer: No.

ECG Abnormalities (%)

History	STØ TØ	ST− TØ	STØ T↑↓	ST↑↓ TØ	ST− T↑↓	ST↑↓ T↑↓
No heart attack *and* no NTG use	4	9	12	17	23	39
Either heart attack *or* NTG use (*not both*)	6	14	17	25	32	51
Both heart attack *and* NTG use	10	20	25	35	43	62

Key to ECG abnormalities (must be in two leads, excluding aVR): ST− = ST-segment "straightening," ST↑↓ = ST segment elevated at least 1 mm or depressed at least 1 mm; T↑↓ = T wave "hyperacute" (>50% of R wave) or inverted at least 1 mm; STØ/TØ = above-specified changes absent.
Directions: To determine a given patient's probability of acute ischemia, start by answering the questions at the top of the chart about the presence of chest pain and whether or not it is the chief complaint. This will lead to one of the three large boxes of probability values. Under the History heading are questions regarding history of heart attack or nitroglycerine (NTG) use. Choose the row that corresponds to the patient's report of none, one, or both of these historical features. Then to find the specific probability value, move across the appropriate row to the column corresponding to the ECG ST-segment and T-wave changes for the given patient. For example, for a patient with a chief complaint of chest pain, no history of heart attack or nitroglycerine use, and 1 mm of ST-segment depression and T-wave inversion, the probability of true ACI would be 78%. (Reproduced from McCarthy BD, Wong JB, Selker HP: Detecting acute cardiac ischemia in the emergency department: A review of the literature. *J Gen Intern Med* 5:365–373. Reprinted with permission of Blackwell Science, Incorporated.)
Note: Specific definitions of clinical features (questions) for original ACI predictive instrument are modified for use in this chart. The original variables were described by Pozen et al. (2).

CRITIQUE
Scientific Basis

The original ACI predictive instrument's predictions are based on a combination of clinical factors using multivariable logistic regression, a mathematical modeling method now commonly used for analogous applications. The outcome predicted—ACI as opposed to AMI alone—matches the emergency physician's task of identifying those patients with unstable angina as well as those with AMI (ie, the entire spectrum of ACI). The clinical variables that the regression uses for its computation are the usual clinical features used by clinicians in assessing the possibility of ACI and include the presence or absence of chest pain or left arm pain/discomfort, chest or left arm discomfort as the most important presenting symptom, history of myocardial infarction, history of use of nitroglycerine for chest pain, ECG ST-segment flattening ("straightening") in two or more leads, ECG ST-segment elevation or depression of 1 mm or greater in two or more leads, and ECG T-wave elevation ("hyperacute") or 1 mm or greater inversion in two or more leads.

The basis for the original ACI predictive instrument's impact on ED care is that the instrument's predicted probability of ACI seems to be incorporated by the physician into ED decisionmaking, especially for patients with lower risk for ACI, and thereby unnecessary (false-positive) hospital and CCU admissions are avoided.

Clinical Practicality

Although the use of a hand-held programmable calculator or a more sophisticated computing system in an ED seems practical, to date the original ACI predictive instrument is not in widespread use, and it may be that a yet more user-friendly mode is needed. A table version of the original ACI predictive instrument has been developed that may be considered more attractive. However, incorporation into computerized electrocardiographs is likely to be the most attractive and practical form.

The original ACI predictive instrument uses some clinical variables that have some room for subjective judgment, particularly for the ECG variables. This is surmounted largely by incorporation of the instrument into modern self-interpreting computerized electrocardiographs in the case of the ACI-TIPI version.

Data from Prospective Clinical Trials in the ED Setting

Studies of Test Sensitivity and Specificity: The diagnostic performance of the original ACI predictive instrument *independent of its use by physicians* has been published (3). However, it is the original investigators' judgment that the tool's predictions should not be used in isolation but only in conjunction with clinical judgment to supplement, not replace, physicians' judgments. Therefore there is no specific probability cutpoint in isolation that corresponds directly to a specific triage decision. Nonetheless, when tested on a separate set of prospectively collected data at the six original study hospitals (N = 2,320), its ROC curve (Figure 7-2) area was 0.89, reflecting excellent diagnostic performance (3). Although for a continuous scale such as 0% to 100% probability, ROC curve area is a much more appropriate measure of diagnostic performance than sensitivity and specificity (which require picking a single cutpoint and ignoring all other information provided by the scale above or below that point). It was noted that the original ACI predictive instrument's ROC curve included the point describing the physicians' diagnostic performance for ACI in the same patients (Figure 7-2), corresponding to a sensitivity of 95% and a specificity of 73%.

The data pertaining to the diagnostic performance of the original ACI predictive instrument were published with the results of the initial ACI-TIPI study (3). When the original ACI predictive instrument's performance was compared with that of the newer ACI-TIPI, their ROC areas were essentially identical (0.89 and 0.88, respectively). For those patients who proved *not* to have ACI, the mean predicted probability of ACI was 24%, and for those who proved to *have* ACI, the average predicted probability was 62% (59% for those with unstable angina, 65% for those with AMI), confirming excellent discrimination.

Studies of the Clinical Impact of the Test's Actual Use: As indicated above, two prospective clinical trials, which included several thousand patients in a wide variety of hospital settings, have provided data that indicate the instrument's safety and effectiveness: the Boston City Hospital (1) and the multicenter (2) trials. The Boston City Hospital study was the pilot study for the larger study and had essentially the same results; thus, only the multicenter trial's results are reviewed here.

As described above, in phase 1, the original ACI predictive

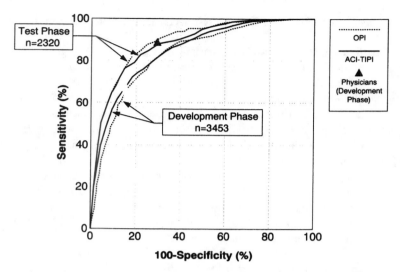

Figure 7-2 Diagnostic performance of the ACI time-insensitive predictive instrument and the original ACI predictive instrument by ROC curves. (Reproduced by permission from Selker HP, Griffith JL, D'Agostino RB. A tool for judging coronary care unit admission appropriateness, valid for both real-time and retrospective use. *Med Care* **1991;29:610. Copyright © 1991 by Lippincott.)**

instrument was developed on the basis of data on the 2,801 study subjects seen in the six participating hospitals. Phase 2 was an 11-month prospective trial of the original ACI predictive instrument's impact. Although it was a prospective controlled clinical trial, patient-by-patient randomization was not used for logistic reasons. Rather, three hospitals had alternating months of intervention/control periods, which avoided threats to validity resulting from changes in physicians or the environment over time; the other three used an experimental/control time-series design, designed to detect any "learning" effect that remained after the switch to "control."

The predictive instrument's use markedly improved physicians' *diagnostic performance*. Specificity was significantly superior during the experimental periods ($P = 0.002$), with no significant change in sensitivity. The false-positive diagnosis ("predictive") rate improved significantly ($P = 0.004$), whereas the false-negative diagnosis rate did not change.

In terms of actual *admission practices*, for patients who proved to have ACI, there was no difference between the experimental and control periods. However, for patients *without* ACI, CCU admission rates were significantly lower during the experimental periods ($P = 0.003$), dropping from 24% to 17% during the control periods. Their ED discharge rates to home increased from 44% during the control periods to 51%. This represents a 30% reduction in CCU admissions for patients without ACI. Using the CCU population as the denominator, the proportion of patients admitted to the CCU without ACI fell from 44% to 33% ($P = 0.001$).

Further analysis was done to try to determine which patients benefited the most from use of the original ACI predictive instrument. For patients whose likelihood of having ACI was less than 50%, there was a 22% reduction ($P = 0.0002$) in the false-positive diagnosis rate during the experimental periods, whereas for patients with a likelihood of having ACI exceeding 50%, the improvement did not reach statistical significance. Thus, the original ACI predictive instrument was most helpful for making a correct diagnosis in patients with less definite signs and symptoms of ACI, whereas physician judgment alone was sufficient to diagnose ACI correctly in patients with higher probabilities of ACI. This is consistent with other results suggesting that much of the original ACI predictive instrument's effect is to reduce uncertainty for the patient for whom the "correct" clinical decision is not clear (5).

Data from Other Clinical Studies

A clinical evaluation in a relatively small sample (N = 243) was reported by Davison et al (6), but its use of the ECG variables was not as intended for the instrument; it divided the scale by cutpoints, and it looked at a different endpoint (complications rather than ACI). Thus it represents a very limited evaluation.

Generalizability to Different Settings

The original ACI predictive instrument has been shown to work in a wide range of hospitals (urban major teaching centers, urban municipal hospitals, teaching affiliates in smaller cities, and rural nonteaching hospitals), and thus, at least for ED use, it seems to be generalizable to different hospital types. Its applicability in other settings has not been directly tested, although given that the variables are relatively unlikely to be directly biased, its applicability to non-ED but related settings seems likely.

In the 1990s, there are now more triage options in some hospitals, such as telemetry and chest pain observation units, than there were in the 1980s. Although the accuracy of the original ACI predictive instrument should not be affected by this, its clinical impact may be different in hospitals with these expanded triage options.

Applicability to Population Subgroups, Including Women and Minorities

The trials of the original ACI predictive instrument included patients from age 30 to 97 years, with a mean age of 62 years and an SD of 14. Unlike the ACI-TIPI, the original ACI predictive instrument has no special handling of the different risks for ACI among women and men, especially over different ages. Nonetheless, no data suggest that this is a problem. Although 92% of subjects in the multicenter trial were white, the fact that the original ACI predictive instrument was shown to be effective at the Boston City Hospital, which has a population with large components of minorities, along with the instrument's similar performance at one other hospital in the multicenter trial with a significant proportion of minority patients, supports the proposition that the instrument is applicable to a variety of patient types.

Cost Considerations

The cost of the use of the original ACI predictive instrument is very low, and its cost implications for overall health care are favorable, as estimated above. An article that looked at the specific cost implications for hospitals in the use of the original ACI predictive instrument pointed out that some projected savings might not be entirely realized because of the cost structure, operations, and incentives inherent in running a hospital (7). Nonetheless, a reduction in unnecessary hospitalizations and CCU stays would presumably be realized, which would produce substantial savings to the system even if the exact size and beneficiary are not yet clear.

Special Concerns

The abovementioned user-friendliness issue should be addressed by use of a computerized electrocardiograph. Given that the ACI-TIPI is implemented in computerized electrocardiographs, it is probably the form of the ACI predictive instruments that will be most widely used (see ACI-TIPI section).

Primary Advantages

The primary advantages of the original ACI predictive instrument are its demonstrated safety and effectiveness in improving ED triage, its low cost, and the high likelihood of improved clinical performance as well as cost benefits (8).

Primary Disadvantages

The issues described above regarding user interface are disadvantages.

SUMMARY AND RECOMMENDATIONS

The original ACI predictive instrument uses readily available clinical and ECG data to compute a probability of ACI. Its diagnostic performance and clinical impact have been well demonstrated in large prospective clinical trials (1,2), which have shown it to be safe and effective in improving ED triage of patients with possible ACI in a wide range of hospitals. Although appropriate for general clinical use, it has not been widely adopted in EDs, possibly because of the need for a hand-held calculator to compute the probability of ACI.

In the near future, the original ACI predictive instrument probably will be superseded by the ACI-TIPI, which may have a similar impact on ED care, with the advantages of computerization and its applicability to retrospective review of care. Since publication of the original ACI predictive instrument trial, ED physicians have become more sophisticated in the triage of patients with ACI. The ACI-TIPI section addresses this further.

Both ACI predictive instruments currently use simple, readily obtained clinical variables. However, neither instrument incorporates the kind of biochemical data that now can be ascertained rapidly in the ED. Modified predictive instruments that incorporate biochemical test data along with data from the clinical history and ECG possibly would be even more powerful instruments, and this approach deserves exploration. Such ACI predictive instruments could provide ways to efficiently use the growing panoply of tests now available (and reviewed in this report) for the evaluation of the ED triage of patients with possible ACI.

The results of the Working Group's final ratings of the quality

Table 7-2   Original ACI Predictive Instrument

ED Diagnostic Performance		ED Clinical Impact	
Quality of Evidence	Accuracy	Quality of Evidence	Impact
A	+++	A	+++

of evidence evaluating this technology and of its ED diagnostic performance and clinical impact are detailed in Table 7-2.

REFERENCES

1. Pozen MW, D'Agostino RB, Mitchell JB, et al. The usefulness of a predictive instrument to reduce inappropriate admissions to the coronary care unit. *Ann Intern Med* 1980;92:238–242.

2. Pozen MW, D'Agostino RB, Selker HP, et al. A predictive instrument to improve coronary-care-unit admission practices in acute ischemic heart disease. *N Engl J Med* 1984;310:1273–1278.

3. Selker HP, Griffith JL, D'Agostino RB. A tool for judging coronary care unit admission appropriateness, valid for both real-time and retrospective use. A time-insensitive predictive instrument (TIPI) for acute cardiac ischemia: a multicenter study. *Med Care* 1991;29:610–627, erratum 1992;30:188.

4. Selker HP, D'Agostino RB, Laks MM. A predictive instrument for acute ischemic heart disease to improve coronary care unit admission practices: a potential on-line tool in a computerized electrocardiograph. *J Electrocardiol* 1988;21:S11–S17.

5. McNutt RA, Selker HP. How did the acute ischemic heart disease predictive instrument reduce unnecessary coronary care unit admissions? *Med Decis Making* 1988;8:90–94.

6. Davison G, Suchman AL, Goldstein BJ. Reducing unnecessary coronary care unit admissions: a comparison of three decision aids. *J Gen Intern Med* 1990;5:474–479.

7. Holthof B, Selker HP. A cost-savings analysis of the use of a predictive instrument for coronary-care-unit admission decisions: a projection of potential national savings based on hospital costs. *Health Care Manage Rev* 1992;17:45–50.

8. Selker HP. Coronary care unit triage decision aids: how do we know when they work? *Am J Med* 1989;87:491–493.

Acute Cardiac Ischemia
Time-Insensitive
Predictive Instrument
(ACI-TIPI)

8

SUMMARY OF TECHNOLOGY

The ACI time-insensitive predictive instrument (ACI-TIPI) represents the next generation of ACI predictive models developed by Selker and colleagues (1,2). The ACI-TIPI improves over the original ACI predictive instrument in two dimensions. First, the tool is incorporated into an electrocardiograph so that its probability predictions are automatically provided along with the conventional 12-lead ECG. Second, the tool is "time insensitive," so it can, as a *single* tool, serve *both* prospective and retrospective purposes. Previously, tools designed for real-time use, such as the original ACI predictive instrument (3), were not validated for retrospective medical record review. Conversely, tools for retrospective review of clinical practice were not applicable to the real-time clinical setting, thus limiting clinicians' interest and confidence in such methods. Thus the time-insensitive predictive instrument (TIPI) was developed to be valid for *both* prospective real-time clinical use and retrospective medical record review to accurately predict a patient's likelihood of having ACI as of the time of ED presentation (1). A potentially useful tool for clinicians, hospital administrators, and payers, it was intended that the TIPI have the added benefit of promoting cooperation between these groups in optimizing CCU use.

In addition to reformulating the original ACI predictive instrument using a new set of clinical variables that could be obtained equally well retrospectively from the medical record and in real time, the ACI-TIPI model includes greater detail in its ECG variables because it was understood that it would likely be incorporated into a computerized electrocardiograph, which would obviate the difficulty of acquiring detailed measurements by physician reading.

In doing so, because of the potential ambiguity of the ECG reading of the "ST-segment straightening" variable in the original ACI predictive instrument, that variable was eliminated in the reformulated instrument. Also, during its reformulation an intentional change was made in the performance of the instrument. Although an instrument for CCU admission should properly identify all patients with ACI (and hopefully thereby help prevent progression to AMI in some), the new instrument was designed to give somewhat higher probability predictions for patients with AMI than for those with unstable angina pectoris, to create bias against false-negative predictions for the more severe cases. This was accomplished by including more detail in the ACI-TIPI's specification of its ECG ST-segment and T-wave variables. For example, in the new instrument, ST-segment depression of 0.1 mV is given one point, depression of 0.2 mV is given two points, and so on, whereas the former instrument merely dichotomized as yes or no for depression of 0.1 mV or more (1).

Specifically, the variables used for the ACI-TIPI are: 1) age, 2) sex, 3) the presence or absence of chest pain or pressure or left arm pain, 4) whether chest pain or pressure is the patient's most important presenting symptom, 5) the presence or absence of ECG Q waves, 6) the presence and degree of ECG ST-segment elevation or depression, and 7) the presence and degree of ECG T-wave elevation or inversion.

The diagnostic performance test phase applied the ACI-TIPI (and the original ACI predictive instrument) to the 2,320 patients seen at the six study hospitals' EDs during the second year. This allowed direct comparison, the results of which are reviewed below. In addition to assessment for its patient-specific predictions, in this phase, there was also testing of specific risk groups based on their "low," "medium," and "high" probabilities of ACI as a potentially more useful output, especially for retrospective review (also see below). In both its patient-based and risk group–based diagnostic performance, the ACI-TIPI showed excellent performance equivalent to the original ACI predictive instrument.

Because the original ACI predictive instrument's requirement for a calculator or chart (see Table 7-1) to generate predictions has limited the instrument's use, as indicated above, the ACI-TIPI was designed to have a more user-friendly form: integrated into a computerized electrocardiograph. Once the non–ECG clinical variables (age, sex, chest pain) have been entered, the machine can compute a patient's probability of having ACI while generating the ECG (2,4). The probability of ACI is then automatically printed on the ECG header to assist the physician's real-time triage decision-making (Figure 8-1). Because conventional computerized electrocardiographs have standard PC microprocessors, the ACI-TIPI's probability data, ECG data, and other information entered directly into the electrocardiograph in clinical use (eg, presenting complaint, age, sex) can be directly transferred to a standard PC, where they can be combined with other data and used for reports and analyses. Combining these tools allows the clinician and operations personnel of a hospital (and payers, health maintenance organizations, malpractice carriers, monitoring agencies, etc) to use the same clinically valid risk-adjusted outcome prediction/measure with no need for separate medical record–based data acquisition.

Given the near-identical performance of the original ACI predictive instrument and the newer ACI-TIPI instrument (1), their use should be considered equivalent. Given its slightly higher scores for patients with AMI, on average, the ACI-TIPI should have a slightly higher sensitivity for AMI (1). The missed AMI rate may be further improved by the incorporation of the ACI-TIPI into an electrocardiograph (2,4), given that a significant contributor to missed AMI in the ED is the misinterpretation of the ECG by the physician (5), which should be diminished by the ACI-TIPI's direct use of the computerized electrocardiograph's ECG variables' measurements (4). The results of early studies have suggested that it has comparable diagnostic accuracy to the original ACI predictive instrument and have shown encouraging impact on ED care (4,6). These latter studies are now reinforced by the recent positive results reported from the 10,689-patient, 10-hospital ACI-TIPI clinical trial, still published only in abstract form (7–9). Finally, in settings where retrospective review of CCU admission practice is desired, the ACI-TIPI, in contrast to the original ACI predictive instrument, is the appropriate technology.

CRITIQUE
Scientific Basis

Like the original ACI predictive instrument, the basis of the ACI-TIPI's prediction is the use of commonly accepted clinical factors

3324561   07/16/1995   06:34:41   AM   JOHN DOE   168 lbs   BP:142/88
                 54 years   Male

Dx: Chest pain chief complaint

Rate   60   : ACI-TIPI PREDICTED PROBABILITY OF ACUTE CARDIAC ISCHEMIA = 91%, based on:
PR   132   : . . Patient is male, age greater than 50
QRSD   94   : . . Patient has chief complaint of chest pain/discomfort or left arm pain
QT   351   : . . No significant Q waves detected
QTc   351   : . . Anterior ST elevation of 0.2 mV or more in two or more of leads V1-V4
               : . . Inferior T waves flat or slightly inverted in two or more of II, III, aVF
— AXIS —   : ACI-TIPI PROBABILITY MAY ASSIST PHYSICIAN TRIAGE JUDGMENT (1.0111 5.1102 9.0050)
P   51
QRS   -36
T   60   PRELIMINARY – MD MUST REVIEW   Edited

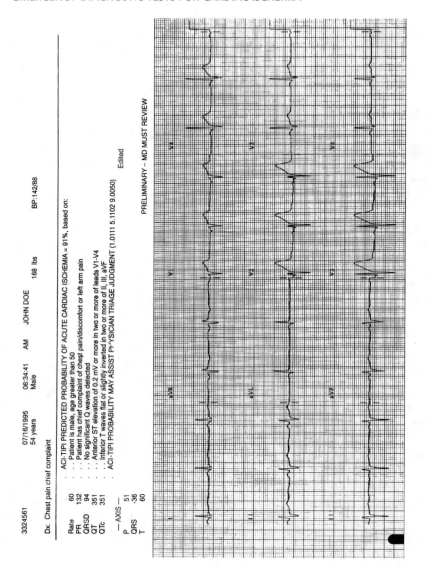

using a mathematical modeling/prediction method widely used for analogous applications. The outcome predicted, ACI, as opposed to AMI alone, seems appropriate to the ED physician's task of identifying those patients with unstable angina as well as those with AMI.

Clinical Practicality

With the caveat mentioned above that the results of the just-completed ACI-TIPI clinical trial should be reviewed in their peer-reviewed published form before a final recommendation, it appears that the ACI-TIPI electrocardiograph is a practical and user-friendly tool for supplementing ED physician triage judgments.

Data from Prospective Clinical Trials in the ED Setting

Studies of Test Sensitivity and Specificity: In the diagnostic performance test phase of the ACI-TIPI study, the ACI-TIPI was tested on prospectively collected data on the 2,320 patients seen at the six study hospitals' EDs during the second year (4). The original ACI predictive instrument was also applied to these patients, allowing direct comparison, and ED physician diagnostic performance for ACI was assessed for comparison to the instruments' predictions. Diagnostic performance was measured by calibration curves, comparisons to final diagnoses, and testing for ability to be unbiased by triage disposition and other features, all of which showed excellent performance. The mean predicted probability for patients who proved not to have ACI was 21%; for those who proved to have ACI, mean predicted probability was 59% (50% for those with unstable angina pectoris and 65% for those with AMI). Calculation of the ROC curve area, which simultaneously evaluates sensitivity and specificity of a continuous scale test, yielded

◀—————————————————————————————

Figure 8-1   ACI time-insensitive predictive instrument.

values of 0.88 to 0.89 for both the ACI-TIPI and the original ACI predictive instrument, demonstrating excellent and very similar diagnostic performance by both (Figure 8-2).

Of interest, the instruments' ROC curve paths include the point depicting ED physicians' performance in their real-time care of the same patients, corresponding to sensitivity of 95% and specificity of 73%. This suggests that the instruments perform comparably to physicians when one considers the probability scale as only "yes" or "no" diagnoses based on a single cutpoint (at probability 25%). Using such a single cutpoint classifies all scores above (and all scores below) the cutpoint as being equivalent. Using such a cutpoint, a 30% probability of ACI is considered diagnostically identical to a 95% probability, and a 20% prediction is considered to mean the same as a 5% prediction; thus much of the clinical information contained in the instruments' 0% to 100% probability scale is lost. Although direct comparison to physicians' performance is not possible, as reflected in the ROC diagram, its performance appears to be comparable. This is quite encouraging for a single

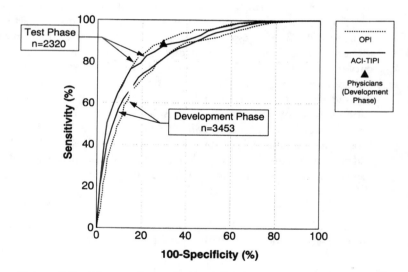

Figure 8-2 Diagnostic performance of the ACI time-insensitive predictive instrument and the original ACI predictive instrument by ROC curves. (Reproduced by permission from Selker HP, Griffith JL, D'Agostino RB. A tool for judging coronary care unit admission appropriateness, valid for both real-time and retrospective use. *Med Care* **1991;29:610. Copyright © 1991 by Lippincott.)**

equation based on a patient's age, sex, complaint of chest pain, and ECG Q waves, ST segments, and T waves.

Although a 0% to 100% probability value such as generated by the ACI-TIPI has more information, and for groups of patients will predict more accurately than dichotomous or categorical diagnoses, in the clinical and especially the retrospective setting there is use for specified probability cutpoints that separate patients into different risk groups. In the ED, the terms "low," "medium," and "high" probability of ACI might be more helpful to some physicians than an actual probability value. Also, for clinical reports, the ability to track risk strata would be helpful. To develop such a risk-stratification system, in the ACI-TIPI's development phase, the 3,453 ED patients were divided into four similar-sized groups based on the ACI-TIPI probability scale, by cutting at 10%, 25%, and 55%, thereby creating higher and lower ACI probability groups. When this was done, the actual midpoint of each probability range, 5%, 17.5%, 40%, and 77.5%, never differed by more than 1% from the actual observed proportion of patients with ACI, a demonstration of the excellent calibration of ACI-TIPI's predictions (1). Given that such low-, medium-, and high-probability groups might be used by themselves as a diagnostic tool, like any other diagnostic test, such categories should be developed on one set of patients and then prospectively tested on an independent sample.

When the performance of the four ACI probability groups was prospectively tested on year 2 patients, among the 552 patients in the low-probability group, only 1.6% had ACI, of whom only 0.7% had AMIs, whereas among the 484 patients in the high-probability group 81.6% had ACI, including 53.3% with AMIs. Of note, as a result of intentional bias built into the ACI-TIPI to give higher scores to ACI patients who had AMI than to those with unstable angina, of those with ACI in each group the subproportions of those with AMI were disproportionately low in the lower-probability groups and disproportionately high in the higher-risk groups. The marked clinical difference between the high- and low-probability groups can be illustrated by comparing them with current ED triage practice. If the entire high-probability group was admitted to the CCU, this would reflect diagnostic performance superior to that of current CCU admitting practices. If all patients in the low-probability group were sent home, fewer patients would be sent home with ACI or AMI (1). In the recent ACI-TIPI trial (7–9), these risk groups were again tested and were again found to have excellent diagnostic discrimination (9).

Studies of the Clinical Impact of the Test's Actual Use: As indicated directly above, the performance of the ACI-TIPI and the original ACI predictive instrument are so similar that it is likely that the results of the prospective controlled interventional trial of the original ACI predictive instrument (3) (described elsewhere in this report) can be considered to apply directly to the ACI-TIPI (1). Although this is likely valid, to confirm this and to examine the impact of the instrument in the current spectrum of intensities of care for triage that were not as available at the time of the original trial, several prospective clinical trials, including a recent large multicenter clinical trial of the ACI-TIPI, have been conducted (7–9).

A small prospective study of 189 patients seen in the UCLA–Harbor Medical Center ED focused particularly on the detection of AMI (4). The ACI-TIPI's results were provided to the ED physicians only after they stated their triage intent, and it appeared that several patients with otherwise missed AMIs were detected by the ACI-TIPI electrocardiograph and were therefore not sent home. This study compared the ACI-TIPI's and physicians' ability to identify patients who proved to have AMI and complications of AMI (defined as the occurrence of life-threatening ventricular arrhythmias and congestive heart failure requiring continuous IV infusion and intensive care). When compared with the physicians' probability estimates, the ACI-TIPI did considerably better both by ROC curve area (0.85 versus 0.64) and when the investigators calculated sensitivity and specificity for the ACI-TIPI by using a previously determined cutpoint of 37%. The ACI-TIPI had a sensitivity for identifying AMI/complication of 93%, specificity of 74%, positive predictive value of 59%, and a negative predictive value of 96%. Physician triage for AMI and/or complications had a sensitivity of 83%, specificity of 69%, a positive predictive value of 52%, and a negative predictive value of 91%.

Although encouraging, this study, a single-blinded study of a sample of convenience, will need confirmation by a prospective clinical trial that tests whether these findings relate to a truly salutary impact of the ACI-TIPI. Also, in this investigation the primary interest was in AMI and complications of AMI, not ACI itself, the outcome for which the instrument was originally intended, and the instrument was used with a "cutoff" score, which has been explicitly avoided as an approach for real-time use by the developers of the ACI-TIPI. These specific issues also will need further investigation.

A study of 605 patients at the University of Geneva (Switzerland) Hospital looked at the possible impact of the ACI-TIPI electrocardiograph on the speed of triage for patients with suspected ACI (6). This hospital's practice is to hold patients in the ED until multiple CK tests are done to confirm the presence of an AMI before CCU admission. This ED practice has two results: 1) There are fewer than half as many false-positive (non-ACI) CCU admissions as are typical of American hospitals, and 2) patients spend much more time in the ED. Thus this trial was not as much directed at changing ED triage *disposition* as it was at changing ED triage *speed*. The question was whether the additional information provided by the ACI-TIPI's probability value would prompt ED physicians and others involved in the care of a patient to triage more quickly.

During this 7-month clinical trial, in the four alternating-month experimental periods, the computerized electrocardiograph printed the ACI-TIPI probability of ACI at the top of all subjects' ECGs. During the 3 control months, the probability was not provided. During the experimental periods, for patients seen by physicians in their first ED rotation, the use of the ACI-TIPI decreased ED time to triage by 0.7 hours (19%, $P = 0.007$). Analyses by type of ACI revealed that the ACI-TIPI's use was associated with a 0.9-hour (25%) reduction for patients with unstable angina ($P = 0.01$), a 0.6-hour (15%) reduction for patients with AMI ($P = 0.1$), and a 1.1-hour (48%) reduction for patients who received thrombolytic therapy ($P = 0.2$). The ACI-TIPI and control groups had no differences in triage appropriateness or mortality. In addition to the ACI-TIPI, important predictors increasing ED time to triage were: 1) patient's age greater than 65 ($+0.9$ hour, $P = 0.0001$), 2) whether the CCU was full ($+0.5$ hour, $P = 0.05$), 3) nighttime ED presentation ($+0.8$ hour, $P = 0.0005$), and 4) thrombolytic therapy use (-1.7 hours, $P = 0.0001$).

As reviewed above, one small (N = 189) and one moderate-sized (N = 605) prospective clinical trials have been conducted, and a large (N = 10,689) multicenter controlled clinical trial was just finished. The data from the first trial (4) suggest that the ACI-TIPI is safe in use, but an exact estimate of its impact on triage was not clear. In the second study (6), a controlled prospective ED trial, there was a specific salutary effect observed (see above) on triage time and on improving the performance of trainees, but the Geneva, Switzerland, setting may not be generalizable to the US situation. Given the very close similarity of the original and newer

ACI predictive instruments (1), it may be that the ACI-TIPI's impact and safety already have been effectively demonstrated, given that the *original* ACI predictive instrument's safety and effectiveness were shown in large clinical trials that included several thousand patients in a wide variety of hospital settings (3,10). Nonetheless, a more comprehensive test of the ACI-TIPI's impact was the goal of the recently finished ACI-TIPI clinical trial (7–9).

The results of the 10,689-patient ACI-TIPI trial showed the diagnostic performance of the ACI-TIPI electrocardiograph by itself and by ACI-TIPI risk groups to be very good (8,9) and showed that its use improved patient ED triage (7).

In terms of its actual impact on ED care, for patients *without* ACI in hospitals with low telemetry capacities, the use of the ACI-TIPI decreased CCU admissions by 16% and increased ED discharge home by 7% ($P = 0.09$). Moreover, for patients seen by residents without supervising attending physicians, the ACI-TIPI's use reduced CCU admissions by 31%, reduced telemetry admissions by 19%, and increased discharged home by 18% ($P = 0.005$).

For patients with stable angina pectoris, in hospitals with *low* telemetry bed capacities, the ED use of the ACI-TIPI reduced CCU admission by 50%, increased telemetry admissions by 25%, and increased ED discharges home by 10% ($P = 0.04$). At hospitals with *high* telemetry capacities, the use of the ACI-TIPI reduced telemetry admissions by 14% and increased ED discharges home by 101% ($P = 0.03$) (the level of discharge seen in hospitals with lower telemetry unit capacities). Across all hospitals, the ACI-TIPI reduced CCU admission by 26% and increased ED discharges to home by 48% ($P = 0.04$).

Finally, for patients with AMI or unstable angina pectoris, at both the low- and high-capacity hospitals, and with both supervised and unsupervised residents, the ACI-TIPI's ED use did not change the appropriate admission of 96% of patients to either CCU or telemetry beds.

Thus, on the basis of this large multicenter prospective controlled clinical trial, if its full report is published as a peer-reviewed article, it would seem that the ACI-TIPI electrocardiograph appears to be safe and effective in a range of ED settings. If so, its use should cause substantial safe reductions in CCU, telemetry, and hospital admissions. The potential additional benefit of using the ACI-TIPI *both* as a real-time ED decision aid *and* as retrospective feedback deserves further investigation.

Data from Other Clinical Studies

A study by Long et al (11) compared the performance of the ACI-TIPI with a recursive partitioning/induced decision-tree method (ID3) to discern the relative advantages of logistic-regression and decision-tree approaches. The ID3 model was developed on the same prospectively collected six-hospital, 3,453-patient data set used to create the ACI-TIPI. When tested on the same test set used for the ACI-TIPI (prospectively collected data on 2,320 ED patients at the six hospitals), its performance was very good (ROC area = 0.82). However, even though it used more variables, its performance was not as good as the ACI-TIPI (ROC area = 0.89) and it had particularly worse calibration. Another comparison by Selker et al (12) between the ACI-TIPI and a neural-network model based on the same data showed initially slightly higher ROC areas for the neural network, but it had more deterioration on the test set and had far worse calibration than the ACI-TIPI. These results reinforce the choice of logistic-regression modeling method used for the ACI-TIPI.

Generalizability to Different Settings

The original instrument was shown to work in a range of different hospital types in its multicenter trial, and the ACI-TIPI was found to be essentially equivalent to the original in the test mentioned above. Thus it too would be expected to be generalizable to EDs in different hospital types. Nonetheless, when available, the results of the ACI-TIPI trial should be reviewed for further information on its generalizability.

Because the ACI-TIPI is typically used in a form in which it is integrated into a computerized electrocardiograph, with the increase in use of the standard 12-lead electrocardiograph in the EMS setting there is the potential for use of the ACI-TIPI in the prehospital setting. An evaluation of the ACI-TIPI's use in the prehospital setting was recently performed by assessing the ACI-TIPI electrocardiograph's performance on ECGs collected in EMS runs, which demonstrated performance in EMS patients equivalent to that seen in ED patients (13). Given these early data, and that patients with chest pain or symptoms suggestive of ACI being transported to the ED should be quite similar to all ED patients with the same complaints, the applicability of the ACI-TIPI to such EMS patients seems reasonable. However, the actual impact of the use of the ACI-TIPI in the EMS setting remains unknown until a prospective interventional clinical trial is done.

Applicability to Population Subgroups, Including Women and Minorities

The ACI-TIPI includes age, sex, and a variable that reflects the interaction of age and sex in the likelihood of ACI. Thus its predictive performance should be good for men and women of a wide age range. It does not include a specific variable for race, but it and its predecessor were modeled and tested on study populations that included a range of racial minority groups. Given the largely physiologic basis of its variables, there seems little reason to expect a difference in its applicability to ethnic minorities. This will be able to be tested further in the ACI-TIPI trial, which includes hospitals with large minority populations.

Cost Considerations

The direct costs of using the ACI-TIPI should be negligible. The ACI-TIPI formula and its implementation in an electrocardiograph are in the public domain; its addition to conventional computerized electrocardiographs can be done by loading ACI-TIPI software. The companies now preparing to introduce it are suggesting that it will likely be a one-time small or no-charge software enhancement to their conventional computerized electrocardiographs (typical ED electrocardiograph price is about $10,000). Once it is obtained, the ACI-TIPI will add no significant costs or additional activities to the usual performance of an ECG.

On the basis of the results of the original predictive instrument trial, it can be anticipated that unnecessary CCU and hospital admissions will be reduced by the use of the ACI-TIPI, which will reduce overall health care costs (14). Whether the 30% reduction in such CCU admissions seen in the original ACI predictive instrument's trial will be seen in the ACI-TIPI trial remains to be seen.

If false-negative mistaken ED discharges to home of patients with ACI are reduced by the ACI-TIPI's use, then the direct and indirect costs associated with the 10,000 to 20,000 patients sent home each year in this country (5) (one of the largest current single causes of adult medical care malpractice litigation) would be reduced. Analyses of the ACI-TIPI clinical trial done at major teaching centers did not show this impact, but further related studies are under way.

Special Concerns

The ACI-TIPI formula is in the public domain. Two companies produced the electrocardiographs that were tested in the recently completed ACI-TIPI trial, generating data on their effectiveness and their safety. As of this writing, one company's ACI-TIPI electrocardiograph has received Food and Drug Administration (FDA) approval and is on the market, and the other's is in the FDA review process for release. Presumably some form of demonstrating equivalence and safety, if not direct testing in a prospective trial, would be appropriate for ACI-TIPI electrocardiographs made by other companies.

Primary Advantages

See the section on the original ACI predictive instrument for discussion of the demonstrated safety and effectiveness of the original form of the ACI instrument improving ED triage (10) and the relatively nominal cost of this technology. Also, the technology adds no significant additional time or effort to usual ED triage procedures. Finally, when retrospective analysis of admission performance is desired, the ACI-TIPI should be able to support this as well as an outgrowth of its use in the real-time clinical setting.

Primary Disadvantages

At this writing, the ACI-TIPI is not yet widely available in all brands of electrocardiographs. However, it soon should be produced by multiple manufacturers as it is available without license in the public domain.

SUMMARY AND RECOMMENDATIONS

The ACI-TIPI, like the original ACI predictive instrument, provides the ED physician with the 0% to 100% probability that a given patient truly has ACI to supplement the ED triage decision. Its diagnostic performance has been tested in large studies that included ED (1,4) and EMS (13) patients and has been demonstrated to be diagnostically equivalent to the earlier version (1), except for a slightly higher sensitivity for AMI. Thus clinical use should be comparable to the original ACI predictive instrument (1), with two advantages for clinical use. First, its incorporation into the conventional computerized electrocardiograph allows direct measurement of details of the ECG waveform without the need for physician interpretation, with automatic printing of the ACI probability on the ECG header. Second, its time insensitivity makes it valid for retrospective review and assessment of care, as well as for real-time ED clinical care.

Table 8-1 Acute Cardiac Ischemia Time-Insensitive Predictive Instrument

ED Diagnostic Performance		ED Clinical Impact	
Quality of Evidence	Accuracy	Quality of Evidence	Impact
A	+++	C*	+*

* Abstract and pending reports are not included in the ratings.

Two published early trials have shown impact on the speed and accuracy of ED triage (4,6). Although published only in abstract form, the trial of clinical impact on ED triage decision-making of a 10,689-patient multicenter controlled clinical trial should provide definitive information regarding the impact of the ACI-TIPI. However, because results of abstracts were not considered in arriving at the Working Group's ratings, at this writing, the quality of evidence warrants a C rating and clinical impact a + until re-rating once the trial's results are fully published.

The overall results of the Working Group's final ratings of the quality of evidence evaluating this technology and of its ED diagnostic performance and clinical impact are detailed in Table 8-1.

REFERENCES

1. Selker HP, Griffith JL, D'Agostino RB. A tool for judging coronary care unit admission appropriateness, valid for both real-time and retrospective use. A time-insensitive predictive instrument (TIPI) for acute cardiac ischemia: a multicenter study. *Med Care* 1991;29:610–627, erratum 1992;30:188.
2. Selker HP, D'Agostino RB, Laks MM. A predictive instrument for acute ischemic heart disease to improve coronary care unit admission practices: a potential on-line tool in a computerized electrocardiograph. *J Electrocardiol* 1988;21(suppl):S11–S17.
3. Pozen MW, D'Agostino RB, Selker HP, et al. A predictive instrument to improve coronary-care-unit admission practices in acute ischemic heart disease: a prospective multicenter clinical trial. *N Engl J Med* 1984;310:1273–1278.

4. Cairns CB, Niemann JT, Selker HP, et al. A computerized version of the time-insensitive predictive instrument: use of the Q wave, ST segment, T wave and patient history in the diagnosis of acute myocardial infarction by the computerized ECG. *J Electrocardiol* 1992;24(suppl):S46–S49.

5. McCarthy BD, Beshansky JR, D'Agostino RB, et al. Missed diagnoses of acute myocardial infarction in the emergency department: results from a multicenter study. *Amm Emerg Med* 1993;22:579–582.

6. Sarasin FP, Reymond JM, Griffith JL, et al. Impact of the acute cardiac ischemia time-insensitive predictive instrument (ACI-TIPI) on the speed of triage decision making for emergency department patients presenting with chest pain: a controlled clinical trial. *J Gen Intern Med* 1994;9:187–194.

7. Selker HP, Beshansky JR, Griffith JL, for the TIPI Working Group. A controlled trial of the acute cardiac ischemia time-insensitive predictive instrument (ACI-TIPI) electrocardiograph on emergency department (ED) triage (abstract). *J Invest Med* 1995;43:497A.

8. Griffith JL, Beshansky JR, Selker HP, for TIPI Working Group. A multicenter prospective test of electrocardiograph–generated ACI-TIPI predictions for acute cardiac ischemia (abstract). *J Invest Med* 1995;43:215A.

9. Griffith JL, Beshansky JR, Selker HP, for TIPI Working Group. A multicenter prospective validation of computerized electro-cardiograph-generated ACI-TIPI risk groups for acute cardiac ischemia (abstract). *J Invest Med* 1995;43:507A.

10. Pozen MW, D'Agostino RB, Mitchell JB, et al. The usefulness of a predictive instrument to reduce inappropriate admissions to the coronary care unit. *Ann Intern Med* 1980;92:238–242.

11. Long WJ, Griffith JL, Selker HP, et al. A comparison of logistic regression to decision tree induction in a medical domain. *Comput Biomed Res* 1993;26:74–97.

12. Selker HP, Griffith JL, Patil S, et al. A comparison of performance of mathematical predictive methods for medical diagnosis: identifying acute cardiac ischemia among emergency department patients. *J Invest Med* 1995;43:468–476.

13. Aufderheide TP, Rowlandson I, Lawrence SW, et al. A test of the acute cardiac ischemia time-insensitive predictive instrument (ACI-TIPI) for prehospital use. *Ann Emerg Med* 1996;27:193–198.

14. Holthof B, Selker HP. A cost-savings analysis of the use of a predictive instrument for coronary-care-unit admission decisions: a projection of potential national savings based on hospital costs. *Health Care Manage Rev* 1992;17:45–50.

Goldman Chest Pain Protocol

9

SUMMARY OF TECHNOLOGY

The Goldman chest pain protocol, a computer-derived decision aid, was developed to assist physicians in using routinely collected clinical and test data in the ED in identifying patients likely to be having an AMI who therefore require triage to the CCU (1). The goal of the original study and follow-up multicenter studies of this protocol was to develop this decision aid and test its likely utility in improving triage to the CCU of patients presenting to the ED with acute chest pain. Because their results were similar, only the larger study is reviewed below.

In the first phase of the multicenter study, the protocol was developed from prospectively collected data on 1,379 patients who presented with acute chest pain to the EDs of two university and four community hospitals. As the outcome to be predicted, on the basis of clinical and test data collected during hospitalization, an AMI was diagnosed if there was one of the following: 1) Characteristic evolution of serum enzyme levels, including a CK–MB fraction of at least 5% of the total CK level, with a typical rise and fall on the quantitative assay, or a level of lactate dehydrogenase isoenzyme 1 that was higher than that of isoenzyme 2 in the absence of hemolysis or renal infarction; 2) ECG development of new pathologic Q waves and at least a 25% decrease in the amplitude of the following R wave, compared with the ECG obtained in the ED; 3) focal uptake of technetium-99 m stannous pyrophosphate on cardiac scintiscan if the serum enzyme peak occurred before hospitalization and if the patient had no history of AMI or valvular calcification; or: 4) sudden unexplained death within 72 hours of ED presentation.

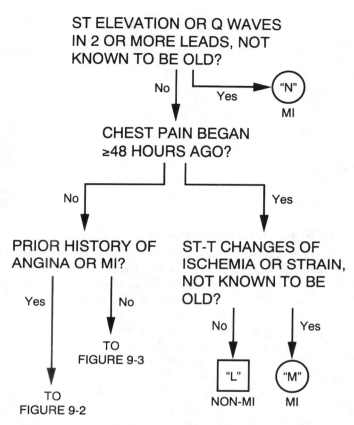

Figure 9-1 Computer protocol for the evaluation of patients with acute chest pain in the ED. The letters "M" and "N" represent groups of patients in whom the predicted probability of acute myocardial infarction (MI) was above 7%, whereas the letter "L" represents a group of patients in whom the predicted probability was less than 7%. If these initial questions do not yield a prediction, the examiner should proceed to either Figure 9-2 (for patients with a history of angina or MI) or Figure 9-3 (for patients with no history of angina or MI). (Reprinted by permission from Goldman L, Cook EF, Brand DA, et al. A computer protocol to predict myocardial infarction in emergency department patients with chest pain. *N Engl J Med* 988;318:797–803. Copyright, 1988 by the Massachusetts Medical Society.)

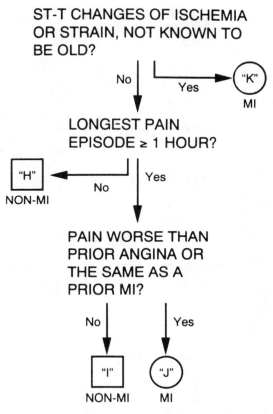

ST-T CHANGES OF ISCHEMIA OR STRAIN, NOT KNOWN TO BE OLD?

No — Yes → "K" MI

LONGEST PAIN EPISODE ≥ 1 HOUR?

"H" NON-MI ← No | Yes

PAIN WORSE THAN PRIOR ANGINA OR THE SAME AS A PRIOR MI?

No | Yes

"I" NON-MI   "J" MI

Figure 9-2 Questions to be asked of patients with a history of angina or myocardial infarction who do not have a new ST-segment elevation or Q waves and whose pain began less than 48 hours previously. The letters "J" and "K" represent groups of patients in whom the predicted probability of acute myocardial infarction (MI) was above 7%; the letters "H" and "I" represent groups of patients in whom the predicted probability was less than 7%. (Reprinted by permission from Goldman L, et al. A computer protocol to predict myocardial infarction in emergency department patients with chest pain. *N Engl J Med* 1988;318: 797–803. Copyright, 1988 by the Massachusetts Medical Society.)

The statistical technique of recursive partitioning was used to divide the study's subjects into subgroups according to certain aspects of the history, physical examination, and ECG, according to whether their proportions of having AMI were higher to lower (Figures 9-1, 9-2, 9-3). The final predictive variables were derived

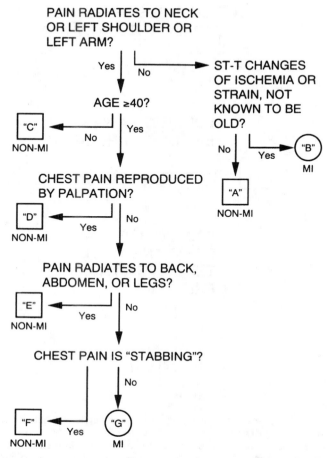

Figure 9-3 Questions to be asked of patients with no history of angina or myocardial infarction and no new ST-segment elevation or Q waves on the ECG whose pain began less than 48 hours previously. The letters "B" and "G" represent groups of patients in whom the predicted probability of acute myocardial infarction (MI) was above 7%, whereas the letters "A" and "C" through "F" represent groups of patients in whom the predicted probability was less than 7%. (Reprinted by permission from Goldman L, Cook EF, Brand DA, et al. A computer protocol to predict myocardial infarction in emergency department patients with chest pain. *N Engl J Med* 1988;318:797–803. Copyright, 1988 by the Massachusetts Medical Society.)

from 50 candidate variables and created 14 groups (labeled with letters "A" through "N", as shown in Figures 9-1, 9-2, and 9-3) based on 9 clinical and 2 ECG features. Admission to the CCU was recommended if the probability of AMI was 7% or higher.

In the second phase of the study, the protocol's diagnostic performance was tested on prospectively collected data from 4,770 patients who presented to the ED with acute chest pain, the results of which are described further below.

CRITIQUE
Scientific Basis

The protocol was developed using prospectively collected data on patients presenting to the ED with acute chest pain. Recursive partitioning was used to develop a decision tree with the probability of ruling in an AMI as the outcome of each branch. The protocol was prospectively validated in a population of 4,770 patients. AMI was used as the outcome on which to base triage to the CCU, given that the risk of emergency complications early in the admission is 17% compared with 5% in patients without AMI.

Clinical Practicality

Given that the sensitivity of the protocol was similar to that of physicians in the likelihood of ruling in for AMI, its greatest utility is in assisting in predicting who will rule out AMI (true negatives), therefore avoiding triage to the CCU. The instrument is easy to use and has been tested as a decision tool in the ED.

Data from Prospective Clinical Trials in the ED Setting

Studies of Test Sensitivity and Specificity: In the primary study of the protocol described above, its diagnostic performance in isolation (ie, not in combination with physician diagnostic judgment other than use of the physician's ECG interpretation) was tested. In the second phase of the study, the protocol's performance was tested on prospectively collected data from 4,770 ED patients who presented with chest pain. Follow-up of the 2,232 patients who were discharged from the ED was performed by physical examination, follow-up measurement of CK, or telephone to determine whether an AMI had occurred after discharge from the ED. Diagnostic performance for AMI compared with that of physicians for the same patients is described in Table 9-1.

Table 9-1 Diagnostic Performance: AMI and Physicians

Parameters	Physicians (%)	Protocol (%)	P
Sensitivity[a]	88	88	NS
Specificity[b]	71	75	<0.00001
Positive predictive value[c]	29	32	0.10
Overall accuracy	73	76	<0.00001

[a] Percentage of patients with AMI admitted to CCU.
[b] Percentage of patients without AMI not admitted to CCU.
[c] Percentage of patients with AMI among the total admitted to CCU.

These data show the sensitivity of the protocol for predicting AMI with triage to the CCU to be the same as that of physicians but with higher specificity than physicians. It was projected that 11.5% of patients without AMI would have been triaged elsewhere had the protocol been used. However, a clinical trial looking for this impact in actual practice from this study was not reported.

Of patients who were not admitted to the CCU but for whom the protocol advised CCU admission, 15% (6 of 41) had a major complication in the 72 hours after ED admission. However, 15% (6 of 40) of patients who were placed in the CCU by the physician for whom the protocol did not advise triage to the CCU had a major complication in the first 72 hours. None of the patients with ACI but not AMI for whom the protocol did not recommend triage to the CCU had a major complication. Of those patients with ACI but without AMI for whom the protocol recommended triage to the CCU and the physician admitted to the CCU, 1.2% (4 of 324) had a major complication in the 72 hours after admission.

Studies of the Clinical Impact of the Test's Actual Use: A prospective trial in which physicians were provided with the protocol used a time-series study design to determine the impact of the protocol on the triage and outcomes of patients presenting to the ED at the Brigham and Women's Hospital in Boston (2). The time-series design used six 14-week cycles, consisting of a 5-week control and/or intervention period separated by 2-week washout cycles. Risk estimates and triage recommendations were provided to physicians in a nonobtrusive fashion. Rates of admissions during intervention and control periods were unchanged in the hospital (52% and 51%, respectively) and in the CCU (10% each). Also, there were no significant differences in hospital length of stay or average total costs (2). Results of prior studies done at the time of the protocol's development have not been reported.

Data from Other Clinical Studies

In another study using the Goldman protocol, Lee et al (3) identified a population with greater than 7% risk of having an AMI in whom a 12-hour the rule-out protocol might be reasonable.

Generalizability to Different Settings

The protocol was developed using data from two urban university hospitals: Yale-New Haven and Brigham and Women's Hospital in Boston (1). Validation of the protocol was performed in these two hospitals and in four community hospitals. The protocol had similar sensitivity and specificity at the university and community hospitals. Therefore it appears that the protocol can be applied to populations in both settings.

Applicability to Population Subgroups, Including Women and Minorities

The training set population was 48% female, and the validation set was 52% female (1). The percentage of racial minorities was not included in the manuscript. Later manuscripts published using the data collected during the validation period reveal that the population presenting with acute chest pain to the Brigham and Women's Hospital was approximately 37% black and 10% Hispanic. Data on race from the University of Cincinnati Hospital revealed that 62% of the patient population presenting to the ED with acute chest pain was black (4). Therefore the protocol was based on a diverse population and should be valid for women and other racial and ethnic groups.

Preliminary data have suggested that blacks are more likely than white patients to present with an AMI *without* chest pain and *with* congestive heart failure (5). It is important to recognize that the protocol addresses patients who present with chest pain.

Cost Considerations

By improving the specificity of physicians' decisions, considerable cost savings may be accrued as a result of triage of patients to less acute, intermediate care beds. It was originally estimated that there could be an $85 million cost savings annually (1).

Special Concerns

Although the protocol's utility in determining the likelihood of AMI appears equivalent to that of physicians, the important issue regarding which patients have unstable angina pectoris (UAP) is not addressed. With the increase in intermediate care units, distinguishing between a very low risk population and those with UAP is important.

The ECG variables used by the protocol include a significant degree of physician skill in reading the ECG. Errors in ECG and/or symptom interpretation could be compounded by the use of the protocol. Results of a prospective controlled clinical trial have not demonstrated its safety and effectiveness in actual clinical use.

Primary Advantages

The protocol's clinical basis is explicit and easy to follow, using routinely obtained clinical and ECG information. The protocol was developed from prospectively collected data and validated in a large population in whom data were also prospectively collected. Diagnostic performance on the test data set was very good. In particular, the protocol has superior specificity in identifying those patients in whom AMI is likely to be ruled out.

Primary Disadvantages

Data from a study prospectively evaluating the actual clinical use of the protocol in an ED suggest little impact on clinical practice (2).

The primary outcome predicted by the protocol is AMI, its focus being triage specifically to the CCU. The protocol does not address the possibility of other forms of ACI, namely, new-onset or UAP.

The protocol evaluates only patients with acute chest pain; its development and testing did not include ED patients who present with primary complaints of shortness of breath, abdominal pain, dizziness, or other symptoms consistent with ACI. Therefore the protocol cannot be considered for patients with possible non-chest pain presentations of ACI, who represent about 24% of all ED patients considered for ACI (6).

SUMMARY AND RECOMMENDATIONS

The Goldman computer-based chest pain protocol was developed using a sound methodology. The fact that it was validated in a large

Table 9-2   Goldman Chest Pain Protocol

ED Diagnostic Performance		ED Clinical Impact	
Quality of Evidence	Accuracy	Quality of Evidence	Impact
A	For AMI: +++ For UAP: NE	B	NK-NE

population that included two university and four community hospitals, with at least two of the hospitals having racially diverse populations, supports its potential utility in a diverse patient population. As the protocol currently stands, its greatest potential benefit would likely be in improving physicians' specificity for AMI and avoidance of triage to the CCU with attendant cost savings. However, this impact has not been demonstrated in a controlled clinical trial of its use. The only published trial of its impact on care suggests that when it is provided to physicians, there is no impact on care and no change in resource utilization (2).

In the time since publication of the protocol, physicians have become more sophisticated in the triage of patients with ACI, and intermediate care units are much more widely used. Thus it would be desirable to see how it classifies patients as they are now triaged in the 1990s. Also, given that UAP may be as important as the possibility of AMI with regard to clinical and cost implications, the fact that non-AMI ACI is not addressed by the Goldman protocol is a significant limitation. Moreover, because non-chest pain presentations of ACI (or AMI) are not considered by the protocol, the protocol may well not be applicable for general identification of ACI among all ED patients with symptoms consistent with ACI. Again, its exact clinical value in current practice settings remains to be demonstrated in interventional clinical trials.

The results of the Working Group's final ratings of the quality of evidence evaluating this technology and of its ED diagnostic performance and clinical impact are given in Table 9-2.

REFERENCES

1. Goldman L, Cook EF, Brand DA, et al. A computer protocol to predict myocardial infarction in emergency department patients with chest pain. *N Engl J Med* 1988;318:797–803.
2. Lee TH, Pearson SD, Johnson PA, et al. Failure of information as an intervention to modify clinical management: a time-series

trial in patients with acute chest pain. *Ann Intern Med* 1995;122: 434–437.

3. Lee TH, Juarez G, Cook EF, et al. Ruling out acute myocardial infarction: a prospective multicenter validation of a 12-hour strategy for patients at low risk. *N Engl J Med* 1991;324:1239–1246.

4. Johnson PA, Lee TH, Cook EF, et al. Effect of race on the presentation and management of patients with acute chest pain. *Ann Intern Med* 1993;118:593–601.

5. Clark LT, Adams-Campbell LL, Maw M, et al. Effects of race on the presenting symtoms of myocardial infarction. *Circulation* 1989;80(4):II–300.

6. Pozen MW, D'Agostino RB, Selker HP, et al. A predictive instrument to improve coronary-care-unit admission practices in acute ischemic heart disease: a prospective multicenter clinical trial. *N Engl J Med* 1984;310:1273–1278.

Other Computer-Based Decision Aids

10

SUMMARY OF TECHNOLOGY

Although the most studied computer-based decision aids for identification of acute cardiac ischemia (ACI) are those described by Pozen et al (1), Goldman et al (2), and Selker et al (3) (all reviewed elsewhere in this report), several other analogous predictive instruments have been described, all for AMI rather than for ACI. These other instruments are reviewed here.

Aase et al (4,5) developed a predictive decision support system (DSP), which uses a bayesian probability model based primarily on historical data, intended to identify patients requiring admission to the CCU as opposed to the general medical ward. Their preliminary data suggest that the DSP also identifies those patients who will ultimately demonstrate verified AMI.

Owing to its growing availability in computer statistical packages and to its general predictive power, logistic regression is the method most commonly used to develop computer-based decision aids for the ED. Tierney et al (6) also developed a logistic-regression model predicting AMI on the basis of history, physical examination, and ECG findings as reported by emergency physicians on a standardized questionnaire. Dilger et al (7) also used logistic regression to predict AMI, using as input variables six variables: cause of admission, duration of pain, leukocytosis, glucose greater than 120 mg/dL, CK greater than 70 IU/L, and ST-segment elevation. Although to some extent each of these decision aids has been evaluated as to its diagnostic performance on patient data (see below), they have not been subjected to a prospective clinical trial of actual use in the real-time clinical setting.

In proposing neural networks as an alternative mathematical

predictive method, Baxt (8) described such a model for predicting presence or absence of AMI in ED patients. The model was developed on a retrospective sample of 351 patients and incorporated 20 input nodes, two hidden layers of 10 nodes each, and a single output node. The actual content of the neural network has not been reported and is apparently considered proprietary. After its development, the neural network was tested on prospectively collected data on 331 patients and showed excellent diagnostic performance (see below). Testing of this model on data from other centers or in actual clinical use has not yet been reported by the original authors. However, a test of this model on an independent data set in a comparison with recursive partitioning and logistic regression showed problems with performance on test data and with calibration.

Although several additional predictive instruments have appeared in the literature, none appears to have been subjected to significant validation or clinical testing. Examples include neural network and recursive partitioning predictive models made using the ACI-TIPI database (9,10). For now, these reports should be considered only preliminary.

CRITIQUE
Scientific Basis

As discussed elsewhere in this document, the clinical/scientific basis for the prediction of AMI as opposed to ACI presents some important limitations to these technologies, which must be kept in mind in reviewing their potential roles.

The authors of the DSP utilized data from 918 consecutive chest pain patients to develop frequency distributions, which were then used to calculate the probability of a particular historical finding given a final diagnosis (AMI, UAP, stable angina pectoris, left ventricular failure, arrhythmia, unspecified chest pain, pulmonary embolism, acute abdominal disease, and miscellaneous disease) (4,5). These same data were used to develop a priori probabilities for the various disease categories. The authors then used these a priori probabilities and symptoms associated with disease categories to calculate posterior probabilities of disease given the patient's symptom complex, using Bayes' formula. They assumed conditional independence among the various symptoms. The derivation set demonstrates a 2 : 1 male/female ratio. No data were provided on minority or age distributions. The authors examined various combinations of historical features (38 characteristics examined) in their model; they do not specify which features were selected for their final predictive model but note that features related to severity and location of pain predominated. Additionally, anxiety and history of coronary heart disease were important in their models.

Tierney et al (6) developed their logistic regression predicting AMI using data on 284 of the 540 patients in their study. Of 22 variables examined, only 4 contributed independent discriminatory power to the model: ECG ST-segment elevation, new pathologic Q waves, diaphoresis with chest pain, and history of AMI. The derived prediction rule was then tested on the remaining 256 patients.

Dilger and colleagues' model (7) included six variables: cause of admission, duration of pain, leukocytosis, glucose greater than 120 mg/dL, CK greater than 70 IU/L, and ECG ST-segment elevation. The model was tested prospectively on 122 patients, as described further below.

Baxt's neural-network model (8) was developed ("trained") on a retrospective sample of 351 patients and incorporated 20 input nodes, two hidden layers of 10 nodes each, and a single output node predicting AMI. The input nodes represented the following clinical variables: age, sex, left anterior location of pain, nausea and vomiting, diaphoresis, syncope, shortness of breath, palpitations, response to nitroglycerine, history of AMI, history of angina, diabetes, hypertension, jugular venous distension, rales, 2 mm ST-segment elevation, 1 mm ST-segment elevation, ST-segment depression, T-wave inversion, and "significant ischemic" changes on ECG. The "trained network" was then tested prospectively on 331 patients, as described below.

Clinical Practicality

Aase's DSP model (4) requires recording numerous historical features; the history protocol has not been administered by ED physicians. The data for the derivation data set and for the prospective study were collected by one of the study authors. At this point, there appear to be insufficient data to judge the applicability of the instrument in usual ED practice.

Tierney and colleagues' model (6) requires only four variables: ECG ST-segment elevation, new pathologic Q waves, diaphoresis with chest pain, and history of AMI. The authors provide coefficients and the constant for their logistic equation; these could be programmed readily into a programmable calculator or portable computer.

Dilger and colleagues' predictive model (7) requires input of six variables: cause of admission, duration of pain, presence or absence of leukocytosis greater than 10,000 μL, blood glucose >120 mg/dL, CK > 70 IU/L, and ECG ST-segment elevation. The authors describe these variables in sufficient detail to allow replication and provide the coefficients and the constant needed to be able to program their logistic regression into a programmable calculator or computer.

Baxt's neural network model (8) is complex and would require a personal computer for use. Additionally, concern about the "black box" nature of a neural network and the lack of having its details published may well limit physician acceptance, despite the promising preliminary results.

Data from Prospective Clinical Trials in the ED Setting

Studies of Test Sensitivity and Specificity: These computer-based decision aids have undergone pilot validation on data from ED settings, with some encouraging results. Unfortunately, these studies have been relatively small, and the instruments have not been tested in other institutions. Until such larger studies in more diverse settings are completed and reported, these reports should be considered preliminary.

The DSP was involved in one prospective study in a single hospital (4,5). The DSP was used to indicate which patients should be admitted to the CCU and which patients were likely to have AMI. Historical data were collected on 1,252 consecutive patients in two phases. During phase I, ED physicians make their admission decisions as usual; in phase II, they used a modified decision protocol using five variables from the DSP. Predictions based on the DSP were generated for patients seen during phase II but were not used in actual patient care decisions. Instead, the DSP's performance was judged on the basis of how decisionmaking would have been influenced had the admission decision actually been based on the DSP's recommendation. When CCU admission decisions were hypothetically made on the basis of the DSP, sensitivity for identifying patients who should go to the CCU was projected at 96%, specificity 56%, positive predictive value 76.5%, negative predictive value 90.4%, and overall accuracy 80%. These values all exceeded those demonstrated by the physicians' usual practice. In differentiating patients with AMI from those with other causes of chest pain, the DSP demonstrated 98.3% sensitivity, 58.9% specificity, 63.1% positive predictive value, 98.2% negative predictive value, and 75.4% overall accuracy. This performance again exceeded that observed in usual ED practice.

As indicated above, Tierney et al (6) developed their predictive model on data from 284 patients and then tested it on their remaining 256 patients. Because the ROC curves developed for the model's performance in both the derivation and validation sets were found to be equivalent, the two portions of their data were recombined, and the ROC area for the whole sample was 0.85. A cutoff probability of 0.10 was advanced by the authors as yielding the best classification performance; model sensitivity was 80.6% (95% CI not reported, but calculated by the reviewer as 78% to 84%). Model specificity was 86% (calculated 95% CI, 83% to 89%), overall accuracy was 85.4% (CI 82.4% to 88.4%), positive predictive value was 43% (CI, 39% to 47%), and negative predictive value was 98% (CI, 97% to 99%).

Dilger et al's predictive model (7) was tested on prospectively collected data on 122 patients, yielding specificity of 86% (95% CI, 80% to 92% by the reviewer's calculation), sensitivity of 89% (calculated 95%, CI 83% to 95%), positive predictive value of 78% (CI, 71% to 85%), negative predictive value of 93% (CI, 88% to 98%), and overall classification accuracy of 87% (CI, 81% to 93%). The authors did not report ROC area or provide information needed for ROC area calculation. The model has not been tested at other centers.

Baxt's neural-network model (8) was tested on prospectively collected data on 331 patients. Using a network output value of 0.55 as the cutoff for diagnosing AMI, the author reported the network's sensitivity as 97.2% (95% CI, 97.2% to 97.5%) and specificity as 96.2% (95% CI, 96.2% to 96.4%). Positive predictive value was not reported but was calculated by the reviewer as 76%, and negative predictive value was calculated by the reviewer as 99.6%. However, its performance showed problems in transportability to test data sets and with calibration when tested by another investigator group (9).

Studies of the Clinical Impact of the Tests' Actual Use: No interventional trial of the real-time clinical use of any of these computer-based decision aids has been reported. Thus it is unknown whether performance would be obtained in actual clinical practice comparable to that found in application to patient data (in isolation from physician input). Moreover, there are no current reports of any of these decision aids currently undergoing clinical trial.

Data from Other Clinical Studies

A study by Long et al (10) compared the performance of a recursive partitioning method, ID3, to the ACI-TIPI (3) logistic regression model in an attempt to discern the relative advantages of the two approaches. Although the ID3 model, developed on the same prospectively collected six-hospital, 3,453-patient data set that was used to create the ACI-TIPI, when tested on the same test set as used for the ACI-TIPI (prospectively collected data on 2,320 ED patients at the six hospitals), its performance was good (ROC area = 0.82) but not as good as that of the ACI-TIPI (ROC area = 0.89). Thus, despite the ID3 model's relatively "competitive" performance and level of testing compared to the decision aids described above, the authors did not propose it for consideration for clinical use. A similar study that included a neural-network model showed it to have ROC areas similar to the ACI-TIPI but poor calibration (9).

Generalizability to Different Settings

The development and single validation study of the DSP have occurred in a single hospital in Norway (4,5). Although the authors indicate that they have some encouraging unpublished data from another hospital, the available report provides no information to assess transportability to other clinical settings. Dilger and colleagues' study (7) was done in Germany, and the other models described above were developed in single hospitals in the United States (6,8–10). As noted above, testing has not been conducted (at least not reported) in settings different from the initial derivation and preliminary validation circumstances. Thus, for all these instruments, generalizability is as of yet unknown.

Applicability to Population Subgroups, Including Women and Minorities

For the DSP, the initial derivation study and the single validation study provide no information regarding minority or age distributions among the patient population used. Additionally, the derivation study population demonstrated a 2 : 1 male/female predominance. At present, these results should be considered preliminary until further validation studies are available demonstrating how this system will function in different settings.

The Tierney et al report (6) indicates that "all males 30 years old and older, and all females 40 years and older" were candidates for their study but does not provide summary descriptive statistics regarding the ultimate sample's characteristics.

For the Dilger et al model (7), 26% of the derivation set were women. The mean age was 60 ± 9 years. The validation set was 33% female. The authors did not describe minority membership in either set. The study took place in western Germany; transportability to heterogeneous populations such as that in the United States was not addressed.

Baxt's study (8) did not report demographics for the training set; the prospective validation set of 331 patients included 192 men (mean age, 51.6 years) and 139 women (mean age, 52.4 years). No further demographic data were provided.

Taken together, these instruments have not yet had sufficient study to ensure applicability to special populations, especially minorities.

Cost Considerations

No specific data are available indicating the potential costs and cost savings that might be accrued by use of any of these instruments.

Special Concerns

General concerns about the paucity of testing and the prediction of AMI rather than ACI are raised above. These proposed decision aids also have a number of special concerns, some of which are described below.

The DSP system depends on the assumption of conditional independence among the variables used in the model. The confidence in the results of the model depends on the underlying assumptions. In this particular model, there are assumptions that the independent variables and/or the sample individuals are not highly related to each other. The results of the analysis might be viewed with some caution. This possibility lends further weight to the need for further validation and then clinical testing.

Dilger et al's model (7) includes CK as one of its predictor variables, in spite of the fact that CK was one of the reference criteria for "gold standard" AMI diagnosis. The authors recognize this potential interdependence of the predictor variable and the reference standard but argue that the model includes only the initial total CK, whereas the reference standard included both CK and CK-MB values measured over 22 hours. Although this probably has only a minor effect on the model's performance, the inclusion of CK might artificially improve the model's performance in this data set, and its variable availability in the ED setting poses a practical obstacle to this decision aid's use.

Baxt's model (8) is clearly the most complex. Neural networks represent a promising technology for predictive instruments because of their ability to discern inapparent relationships among variables. However, their complexity and the difficulty in defining how they arrive at their predictions present possible impediments to their widespread acceptance. Whereas multivariate logistic regression and recursive partitioning–like models provide explicit information regarding variables' contribution to the model's performance, the relationships among variables in a neural network are "buried" in connection strength and weight matrices, which might appear inscrutable to those not intimately familiar with the model. This concern should not stand in the way of further investigation of these models; we should simply be cognizant of these potential drawbacks. Unfortunately, the fact that Baxt's model was not published or made available in a way that others can validate only reinforces concerns about the opaque "black box" aspect of this approach. Availability for testing by other investigators remains the standard for scientific contributions, and this hurdle will need to be surmounted before acceptance of this decision aid, no matter what performance data are published by its originators. The closest possible test of Baxt's model has shown potential limitations to transportability and calibration (9).

Primary Advantages

The potential of decision aids predicting ACI/AMI to improve care has been demonstrated in publications of the aids that have been more widely tested, and if these models are proved to be safe and effective, similar benefits presumably could be accrued.

Primary Disadvantages

As noted above and discussed elsewhere in this document, the prediction of AMI rather than ACI is a disadvantage.

Additionally, it is unclear just how burdensome data collection might be for some of these other instruments in clinical use. The authors provide little or no information indicating how long data

Table 10-1   Other Computer-Based Decision Aids

ED Diagnostic Performance		ED Clinical Impact	
Quality of Evidence	Accuracy	Quality of Evidence	Impact
B	+	NK	NK

collection for these decision aids might take in real-time use, which could be a significant barrier in the busy clinical setting of the ED with acutely ill patients.

None of these instruments has been shown to be safe and effective in a controlled clinical trial, and it is not clear how these tools should interface with physicians' own judgments. Clearly, at this stage, they are not appropriate for clinical use.

As indicated above, the potentially opaque nature of the workings of these computer-based aids, especially the neural network, remains a barrier to investigation and potentially to clinical acceptance.

The medical-legal implications of the use of these aids also need exploration.

SUMMARY AND RECOMMENDATIONS

These computer-based decision aids provide examples of a variety of ways to identify patients for CCU admission but have a number of major limitations, especially that they predict AMI rather than ACI and have not yet been demonstrated to be safe and effective in actual use. In addition, there are some concerns about the generalizability and transportability of some of their input variables and, for the neural network model of Baxt (8), concerns about the black box and lack of publication of the model to allow testing by others.

Although each of these models has some promise, including very encouraging performance in their preliminary studies, at this point, none can be considered ready for clinical use.

The results of the Working Group's final ratings of the quality of evidence evaluating these technologies and of their ED diagnostic performance and clinical impact are supplied in Table 10-1.

REFERENCES

1. Pozen MW, D'Agostino RB, Selker HP, et al. A predictive instrument to improve coronary-care-unit admission practices

in acute ischemic heart disease: a prospective multicenter clinical trial. *N Engl J Med* 1984;310:1273–1278.

2. Goldman L, Cook EF, Brand DA, et al. A computer protocol to predict myocardial infarction in emergency department patients with chest pain. *N Engl J Med* 1988;318:797–803.

3. Selker HP, Griffith JL, D'Agostino RB. A tool for judging coronary care unit admission appropriateness, valid for both real-time and retrospective use. A time-insensitive predictive instrument (TIPI) for acute cardiac ischemia: a multicenter study. *Med Care* 1991;29:610–627, erratum 1992;30:188.

4. Aase O, Jonsbu J, Liestøl K, et al. Decision support by computer analysis of selected case history variables in the emergency room among patients with acute chest pain. *Eur Heart J* 1993;14:433–440.

5. Jonsbu J, Aase O, Rollag A, et al. Prospective evaluation of an EDB-based diagnostic program to be used in patients admitted to hospital with acute chest pain. *Eur Heart J* 1993;14: 441–446.

6. Tierney WM, Roth BJ, Psaty B, et al. Predictors of myocardial infarction in emergency room patients. *Crit Care Med* 1985;13: 526–531.

7. Dilger J, Pietsch-Breitfeld B, Stein W, et al. Simple computer-assisted diagnosis of acute myocardial infarction in patients with acute thoracic pain. *Methods Inf Med* 1992;31:263–267.

8. Baxt WG. Use of an artificial neural network for the diagnosis of myocardial infarction. *Ann Intern Med* 1991;115:843–888.

9. Selker HP, Griffith JL, Patil S, et al. A comparison of performance of mathematical predictive methods for medical diagnosis: identifying acute cardiac ischemia among emergency department patients. *J Invest Med* 1995;43:468–476.

10. Long WJ, Griffith JL, Selker HP, et al. A comparison of logistic regression to decision tree induction in a medical domain. *Comput Biomed Res* 1993;26:74–97.

Creative Kinase

11

SUMMARY OF TECHNOLOGY

The ECG and a history of chest pain have been the primary methods for screening patients for ACI and AMI (1). Of critical importance, the presenting ECG in the ED may be nondiagnostic in more than 50% of patients. ST-segment elevation on the 12-lead ECG is considered to be strong evidence of an evolving Q-wave AMI in patients with chest pain in the ED and at the center of the decision pathway for reperfusion therapy. Biochemical markers of AMI are of great importance in those patients in whom the ECG is nondiagnostic. Current data do not support the administration of thrombolytic agents to patients with a non–Q-wave AMI, although it remains clinically relevant to identify such patients for admission to the hospital, medical therapy, and possible cardiac catheterization. The best-studied biochemical marker of myocardial necrosis is CK.

CK performs the reversible reaction of converting creatine phosphate and adenosine diphosphate to creatine and adenosine triphosphate. CK isoenzymes are three species of dimers with roughly 60,000-Da molecular weight, composed of combinations of two possible subunits (M, muscle; B, brain). The CK-MM isoform is found mostly in skeletal muscle, whereas CK-BB is found both in kidney and brain tissue. Small amounts of CK-BB may also be synthesized by malignant cells. The myocardium has the highest concentration of CK-MB isoenzyme, but there is roughly four to five times more CK-MM isoenzyme than CK-MB isoenzyme. Thus, for each unit of CK-MB released into the bloodstream, four to five units of CK-MM will also be released. Because CK-MM has a longer half-life than CK-MB, it will continue to be elevated even after CK-MB falls below detectable levels.

There are numerous noncardiac and cardiac causes of total serum CK increase. Most of the noncardiac causes are related to skeletal muscular disease or injury. It should be noted that small amounts of CK-MB can be found in the small intestine, tongue, diaphragm, uterus, and prostate. Some tumors in these organs can produce CK subunits, potentially confounding determination of the source of CK increase. Therefore the arbitrary designation of "normal" reference levels without evaluation of the entire curve and interpretation in the clinical context in which the specimens were obtained can be potentially misleading.

Although AMI is typically associated with elevation of total CK and CK-MB, skeletal muscle damage can also increase total CK and increase CK isoenzymes above the usual 3% to 5% of total CK. "White" skeletal muscle fibers have negligible CK-MB levels, and "red" skeletal muscle fibers contain as much as 10% CK-MB. Factors that increase the numbers of red fibers include physical conditioning and vigorous exercise, and these situations can lead to higher levels of CK-MB release in the circulation.

Techniques for measurement of CK and MB activity are available for both plasma and serum. Common methods of measuring CK-MB include enzymatic activity assays (with results expressed as units per liter) and mass assays (with results expressed as nanograms per milliliter or micrograms per liter). Commonly employed enzymatic activity assays include electrophoretic assays and ion-exchange columns. Newer assays based on monoclonal antibodies that measure CK-MB mass are rapid, highly sensitive, and specific and are becoming the analytic method of choice (2,3). There is some evidence that abnormal levels of CK-MB measured by mass assay may be detected approximately 1 hour earlier than CK-MB measured by activity assay and total CK in the setting of AMI (4).

To increase the specificity of a single CK-MB, it has been suggested that a CK-MB mass/total CK activity index of 2.5 may more accurately differentiate myocardial from skeletal muscle damage, and cutoff values of 2.5 to 3.0 are in common use (5). This range of cutoffs may not be useful for trauma patients with cardiac contusion in whom total CK is greatly increased and a small but significant amount of CK-MB from cardiac muscle may not reach the cutoff. In addition, in chronically injured skeletal muscle, the release of CK-MB may be very large, leading to a decreased specificity of the test with the stated cutoff. Also, an increased CK-MB and index cannot distinguish among AMI, cardiac contusion, electrical injury, and pericarditis. Such determinations need to be made on clinical grounds.

Measurement of CK-MB over a 12- to 24-hour period is currently the test of choice for the diagnosis of AMI. Increases in plasma levels are characteristically seen within 6 to 10 hours of the onset of coronary occlusion and AMI. Peak values are seen at 17 to 24 hours, and levels return to the normal range in approximately 36 to 72 hours. Early (<6 hours after symptoms begin) CK-MB is poorly sensitive. Because a period of 8 to 10 hours is frequently required for plasma levels of CK-MB to become increased in the range that provides a reliable diagnosis of AMI, the potential use of single CK-MB testing as an ED early diagnostic marker appears to be limited.

However, further examination of isoforms of CK-MB can improve the early sensitivity of the test. CK-MB released from myocardial cells into the plasma is acted on by the enzyme carboxypeptidases, which catalyze the loss of a terminal lysine from the C-terminus of the M subunit. The tissue form (CK-MB2 and conversion products) is typically seen in equal concentration with CK-MB1 in the plasma. Diagnosis of AMI by CK isoforms can be made earlier (<4 hours) than that based only on CK-MB increases because the ratio of tissue/circulation isoforms becomes abnormal before CK-MB is increased above the upper limit of normal (6–11). A false-positive finding may occur because CK-MB2 can result from skeletal muscle injury. With this method, it is important to exclude patients with skeletal muscle injury to maintain specificity (12).

Biochemical testing for the diagnosis of AMI is rapidly evolving from the classic enzymatic activity-type assays to mass determinations by immunoassay techniques. New, small, hand-held cassettes for bedside qualitative determinations of CK-MB using specific monoclonal antibodies are undergoing clinical trials. Typically, a patient's blood specimen is placed in a well and applied to a membrane. The membrane separates RBCs from plasma. Highly specific antibodies against CK-MB complex with CK-MB in the plasma and a colored precipitin line are formed usually in less than 20 minutes.

CRITIQUE
Scientific Basis

Serial measurement of CK and CK-MB, for the first 24 hours after presentation to the ED, has high sensitivity (100%) and specificity

(98%) for the detection of AMI (13). The sensitivity and specificity of a single CK/CK-MB was carefully studied by Lee et al (14). The sensitivity of CK-MB, using a CK-MB activity level greater than 5% of total CK, ranges from 25% to 57%, increasing with increasing length of time between onset of symptoms and presentation to the ED. The specificity for AMI of a single CK is approximately 80%. The specificity of a single CK-MB is 88% (false-positive rate, 12%). However, because this study was performed with ion-exchange chromatography measurements for CK-MB, a technology that is less accurate than CK-MB mass, the findings may not apply to current practice. In addition, increased CK-MB returns to normal within 2 to 3 days of myocardial injury, decreasing its utility in patients who present more than 48 hours after the ischemic event.

There are important shortcomings in the use of CK for making a triage decision: The most fundamental problem is that if the patient is having noninfarction ACI, the CK will (by definition) be normal, and yet triage should be appropriate to the presence and potential dangers of UAP, including progression to AMI. Also, even if the patient is having an AMI, the CK can be normal early in its course. Indeed, even if the patient's symptoms of ACI have been present for some time, thrombosis causing AMI itself may not yet or only recently have occurred, in which case the CK would still be normal. This latter issue can be significantly but not completely ameliorated by obtaining CK tests over a period of time, perhaps in the range of at least 6 hours, with additional sensitivity increasing with increases in time to 12 or more hours. The former issue, that of the negative test in noninfarction ACI, cannot be surmounted with CK (or CK-MB) testing.

Clinical Practicality

Most physicians are familiar with measurement of CK and CK-MB and are generally comfortable with interpretation of the results of activity assays, which are measured in international units per liter. Mass measurements use the units nanogram per milliliter. In view of their high specificity for CK-MB, they obviate the need for confirmatory tests such as electrophoretic assays. Because these techniques can be performed rapidly, they facilitate the ability to obtain repeat tests over intermediate periods of time, such as 6 to 12 or more hours.

Data from Prospective Clinical Trials in the ED Setting

Studies of Test Sensitivity and Specificity: The development of immunochemical methods to detect CK-MB has substantially improved the sensitivity of this marker for detecting acute myocardial necrosis. There have been several studies evaluating the utility of CK-MB either as a single test or frequent sampling in the hours after presentation to the ED. In a preliminary study, Gibler and colleagues (13) used serial immunochemical CK-MB analysis to provide early identification of patients with AMI having a nondiagnostic 12-lead ECG on presentation to the ED. Within 3 hours after presentation, sensitivity for the hospital diagnosis of AMI by immunochemical CK-MB assays was approximately 95%. These findings were confirmed in a multicenter prospective trial by the Emergency Medicine Cardiac Research Group (EMCREG) in 616 patients (15). Marin and Teichman (16) developed an algorithm using an initial CK-MB of 10 ng/mL as a cutoff and an additional measurement of CK-MB at 2 hours to achieve a sensitivity of 94% and a specificity of 91% for early detection of AMI. However, follow-up data in this study were obtained in only 78% of the study population. These studies suggest a reconsideration of the older studies, which maintained that CK-MB testing was not a viable diagnostic strategy for the ED. Although reasonable in theory, using CK-MB to effect ED triage of patients still requires prospective validation.

Studies from the 1980s showed the very limited sensitivity and specificity of a single CK or CK-MB test from the ED. These had the effect of discouraging the emergency physician from using the initial CK in making the initial decision to hospitalize or discharge the patient. Viskin et al (17) studied the contribution of measuring serum CK levels to making the diagnosis of AMI in the ED. Among patients presenting within 4 hours of symptoms, the ECG identified 66%, whereas serum CK levels identified only 9%. However, among patients evaluated more than 4 hours from the onset of chest pain, the ECG was useful in the diagnosis of AMI in 36.6%, whereas serum CK levels were increased in 63.4%. When comparing single CK and CK-MB determinations in the ED for diagnosing AMI, Lee et al (14) found that the sensitivities and specificities of both CK and CK-MB were higher in patients presenting more than 4 hours after the onset of symptoms. However, the sensitivity of a single CK or CK-MB sample was too low (34%

to 38%) to exclude the diagnosis of AMI. By using the more accurate CK-MB mass test, and by stratifying on patient time of arrival to the ED, some investigators have argued that an initial positive CK-MB may have some utility in reversing the decision to discharge a patient, some of whom were subsequently demonstrated to have AMI (5,18). This strategy has not been prospectively validated.

One of the largest trials of a new biochemical marker—CK-MB isoforms—in ED patients involved 1,110 patients with chest pain who had blood specimens collected every 30 to 60 minutes for at least 6 hours after the onset of symptoms (19). The diagnosis of AMI was established using quantitative criteria for CK-MB isoforms (MB2 activity of >1.0 U/L and/or a ratio of MB2/MB1 of >1.5). Receiver-operating characteristic (ROC) curves indicated that the CK-MB subform criteria noted above had the optimum performance at 6 hours; sensitivity for AMI was 95.7% and specificity was 93.9%. At 4 hours, sensitivity was 56% and specificity was 93%. However, this study did not ascertain AMI outcomes in discharged patients, and thus the prevalence of disease was higher with a bias toward higher sensitivities for all methods. Given the conversion of MB2 to MB1 and other isoforms, this assay has limited use in patients who present later (more than 24 hours) into the course of their AMI. Also, MB isoforms are subject to the same limitations in specificity as MB. Again, the actual clinical impact of using this assay in a population of patients presenting to an ED with acute chest pain has not been prospectively tested.

Studies of the Clinical Impact of the Test's Actual Use: It also appears that the availability of early serum markers such as CK-MB affects decisionmaking in the emergency setting. In a substudy of the first EMCREG trial (13), the availability of serial CK-MB results appeared to impact decisionmaking in one third of patients presenting to the ED with possible AMI (5). These CK-MB data strengthened physican impression of AMI in patients having AMI and a nondiagnostic 12-lead ECG while decreasing the impression of AMI for non-AMI patients. These results served as a pilot for EMCREG 2 (15), a prospective trial that measured the impact of 0- and 3-hour CK-MB results on emergency physician decisionmaking in 1,042 patients presenting to the ED with a nondiagnostic 12-lead ECG. Again, positive serial CK-MB results tended to confirm physician impression of an evolving AMI, precipitating diposition to an intensive care setting. Alternatively, negative serial

CK–MB results caused the physician to disposition the patient to a non–intensive care bed, or prevented the inappropriate discharge of a small number of patients with AMI (18,20).

Despite these important multicenter studies of the potential impact of CK–MB testing, there has not yet been a similar prospective trial of its actual impact on overall triage on the domain of all ED patients with chest pain or other symptoms suggestive of ACI with follow-up of those triaged home.

Data from Other Clinical Studies

An increase in the initial or 2-hour CK–MB appears to have prognostic value in patients with symptoms suspicious of AMI but with a nondiagnostic ECG. Hoekstra et al (21) demonstrated in a multicenter trial of 5,120 patients that a positive ED CK–MB at 0 or 2 hours was associated with a greatly increased risk of death or hospital complications. This confirmed the results of preliminary work (22).

Clinical studies in non–ED settings have been used to help establish the reference range for the new CK–MB mass assays (23). There have been a number of retrospective studies evaluating the sensitivity and specificity of CK, CK–MB, and MM and MB isoforms in differentiating patients with AMI. A single CK or CK–MB may add little additional information beyond the ECG in patients with AMI (24).

Generalizability to Different Settings

Interpretation of increased CK–MB values can be confounded by the numerous conditions, both cardiac and noncardiac, that can increase this enzyme marker. Specific problems likely to be encountered in the ED include skeletal muscle trauma, cardiac contusion, and pericarditis. Potentially confusing scenarios could develop in patients with hypothyroidism and malignancies, although they are rarely seen.

Applicability to Population Subgroups, Including Women and Minorities: Although slightly different reference ranges may be applicable for CK–MB in whites versus blacks and men versus women, this should not present a significant problem. Single CK or CK–MB measurements that are just above the upper limit of normal for the reference range require additional confirmatory data (as described above). At present, patients are frequently admitted to the hospital to obtain such confirmatory data, but alternative triage

programs such as a coronary observation unit (for approximately 6 to 12 hours) might serve this purpose quite well.

There are few data on the racial makeup of the populations in which the sensitivity and specificity data are based. There have been no analyses specifically addressing the sensitivity and specificity of the enzyme assays in minorities or in women in the ED setting.

Cost Considerations

Sophisticated radioimmunoassays and electrophoretic analyses are time consuming and potentially expensive and require skilled personnel. Although automated analyzers are expensive, the introduction of automated analyzers, particularly those that utilize highly specific antibodies to CK–MB, have the potential for considerable overall cost savings to the health care system. These new automated analyzers can process specimens at a rate of about one specimen every 8 to 15 minutes, can be run in the batch mode, obviate the need for confirmatory tests such as electrophoretic assays, and can potentially shorten hospital stays for "rule-out AMI" cases (11).

Although the costs of performing CK and CK-MB determination may be low, the aggregate cost would not be negligible if used several times on each of the estimated 7 million patients who present yearly to EDs with chest pain or other symptoms consistent with ACI. However, if effective, although more expensive than the use of the standard ECG, its cost would compared quite favorably with imaging technologies and would seem well justified in the context of the potential savings in hospital costs and of mortality and morbidity related to failure to admit ACI patients.

Special Concerns

The high number of potential causes of false-positive increases of total CK and CK-MB could present a diagnostic dilemma in the ED. Given the widespread availability of rapidly obtaining CK and CK-MB determinations in EDs, it is important for physicians to understand the inherent limitations of these data. Reliance on CK and CK-MB data may lead to inappropriate discharge of patients with AMI and ACI. Similarly, inappropriate reliance on CK and CK-MB data may lead to overutilization of resources given the less-than-perfect specificity of the enzyme data.

In view of the delay for CK and CK-MB to become increased above the upper limit of normal and potential confusion with skeletal muscle sources, clinicians cannot rely completely on isolated measurements of CK to confirm the diagnosis of AMI. Supplementary data are essential, such as additional CK measurements (eg, separated by as little as 2 hours) or simultaneous measurement of other serum markers (eg, myoglobin, troponin-I or -T, myosin light chains). Serial CK-MB determinations have superior sensitivity (68%) and specificity (95%) for diagnosis of AMI compared with serial ECG determinations (sensitivity, 39%; specificity, 88%) on inpatients presenting with initially nondiagnostic ECGs (24).

Primary Advantages

There is generally uniform familiarity with CK and CK-MB assays. There is an extensive database from clinical experience with this serum marker in more than four decades of coronary care medicine and ED evaluation of patients with chest pain syndromes. CK and CK-MB data can be obtained quickly in most EDs. For patients in whom the likelihood of AMI is high, a positive value can further strengthen the likelihood of AMI. Serial CK-MB testing is more effective than single CK-MB testing in excluding AMI.

Primary Disadvantages

The primary disadvantage of CK and MB enzyme testing lies in its poor early (<6 hours) and late (>48 to 72 hours) sensitivity. Second, there is some lack of specificity of CK, CK-MB, and MM and MB isoforms as a result of the presence of these enzymes in tissues other than myocardium, but the false-positive rate occurs less than 5% of the time (21). Third, most of the investigations evaluating the utility of these enzymes use AMI as the outcome measure. CK, CK-MB, and MM and MB isoforms have little utility in identifying UAP.

SUMMARY AND RECOMMENDATIONS

CK and CK-MB measurements are traditionally obtained early in the ED course of a patient admitted to the hospital for suspected AMI or ACI. The utility of the assay in the ED as a one-time test is limited because levels do not significantly increase until 4 to 6 hours after the onset of AMI. Mass measurements of CK-MB, compared with the older activity analysis, have improved sensitivity and specificity. Improved sensitivity may also be achieved by CK-MB subforms, and these may be more useful in making the diagnosis of AMI in the ED for patients who present early after the onset

Table 11-1 Creatine Kinase

| | ED Diagnostic Performance | | ED Clinical Impact | |
	Quality of Evidence	Accuracy	Quality of Evidence	Impact
Single test	A	For AMI: + For UAP: NE	NK	NK
Multiple tests over time	A	For AMI: + + + For UAP: NE	NK	NK

of symptoms. This is also achieved by the repeated measurements of CK-MB in the ED or the hospital. However, and importantly, CK and CK-MB do not identify patients with UAP, who constitute about half of patients with ACI.

Despite improvements in the diagnostic performance and practicality of CK and CK-MB assays, there is no controlled clinical impact trial showing that these tests are effective for decisions to send a patient home or to the appropriate level of care of admission for patients with suspected ACI, either as one-time or serial tests. A prospective intervention study, with follow-up of all (including nonadmitted) patients, of the effect of serial CK and CK-MB on patient outcomes is needed before a strategy incorporating CK-MB into medical decisionmaking can be fully evaluated or recommended.

The results of the Working Group's final ratings of the quality of evidence evaluating this technology and of its ED diagnostic performance and clinical impact are shown in Table 11-1.

REFERENCES

1. Lee TH, Cook FE, Weisberg M, et al. Acute chest pain in the emergency room: identification and examination of low risk patients. *Arch Intern Med* 1985;145:65–69.
2. Green GB, Hansen KN, Chan DW, et al. The potential utility of a rapid CK-MB assay in evaluating emergency department patients with possible myocardial infarction. *Ann Emerg Med* 1991;20:954–960.
3. Mair J, Artner-Dworzak E, Dienstl A, et al. Early detection of acute myocardial infarction by measurement of mass concentration of creatine kinase-MB. *Am J Cardiol* 1991;68:1545–1550.

4. Wu AHB, Gornet TG, Harker CC, et al. Role of rapid immunoassays for urgent ("stat") determinations of creatine kinase isoenzyme MB. *Clin Chem* 1989;35:1752–1756.

5. Young GP, Hedges JR, Gibler WB, et al. Do CK-MB results affect chest pain decision making in the emergency department? *Ann Emerg Med* 1991;20:1220–1228.

6. Puleo PR, Guadagno PA, Roberts R, et al. Sensitive, rapid assay of subforms of creatine kinase MB in plasma. *Clin Chem* 1989; 35:1452–1455.

7. Puleo PR, Guadagno PA, Roberts R, et al. Early diagnosis of acute myocardial infarction based on assay for subforms of creatine kinase-MB. *Circulation* 1990;82:759–764.

8. Adams JE, Abendschein DR, Jaffe AS. Biochemical markers of myocardial injury; is MB creatine kinase the choice for the 1990's? *Circulation* 1993;88:750–763.

9. Short SG, Clements SD. What to know about cardiac isoenzymes: an update. *Prim Cardiol* 1993;19(11):55–56, 62–64.

10. Roberts R, Kleiman NS. Earlier diagnosis and treatment of acute myocardial infarction necessitates the need for a "new diagnostic mind-set." *Circulation* 1994;89(2):872–881.

11. Apple FS. Acute myocardial infarction and coronary reperfusion: serum cardiac markers for the 1990s. *Am J Clin Pathol* 1992;97(2):217–226.

12. Wu AH, Wang XM, Gornet TG, et al. Creatine kinase MB isoforms in patients with skeletal muscle injury: ramifications for early detection of acute myocardial infarction. *Clin Chem* 1992; 38(12):2396–2400.

13. Gibler WB, Lewis LM, Erb RE, et al. Early detection of acute myocardial infarction in patients presenting with chest pain and nondiagnostic ECGs: serial CK-MB sampling in the emergency department. *Ann Emerg Med* 1990;19(2):1359–1366, erratum 1991;20(4):420.

14. Lee TH, Weisberg MC, Cook EF, et al. Evaluation of creatine kinase and creatine kinase-MB for diagnosing myocardial infarction; clinical impact in the emergency room. *Arch Intern Med* 1987;147:115–121.

15. Gibler WB, Young GP, Hedges JR, et al. Acute myocardial infarction in chest pain patients with non-diagnostic ECGs: serial CK-MB sampling in the emergency department. *Ann Emerg Med* 1992;21:504–512.

16. Marin MM, Teichman SL. Use of rapid serial sampling of creatine kinase MB for very early detection of myocardial infarc-

tion in patients with acute chest pain. *Am Heart J* 1992;123: 354–361.

17. Viskin S, Heller K, Gheva D, et al. The importance of creatine kinase determination in identifying acute myocardial infarction among patients complaining of chest pain in an emergency room. *Cardiology* 1982;74:100–110.

18. Hedges JR, Gibler WB, Young GP, et al. Multicenter study of creatine kinase-MB use: effect on chest pain clinical decision making. *Acad Emerg Med* 1996;3:7–15.

19. Puleo PR, Mayer D, Wathen C, et al. Use of a rapid assay of subforms of creatine kinase MB to diagnose or rule out acute myocardial infarction. *N Engl J Med* 1994;331:561–566.

20. Gibler WB, Young GP, Hedges JR, et al. Serial CK-MB levels impact physician decision-making in patients presenting to the emergency department with chest pain (abstract). *Med Decis Making* 1992;12(4):332.

21. Hoekstra JW, Hedges JR, Gibler WB, et al. Emergency department CK-MB: a predictor of ischemic complication. *Acad Emerg Med* 1994;1:17–28.

22. Hedges JR, Young GP, Henkel GF, et al. Early CK MB elevations predict ischemic events in stable chest pain patients. *Acad Emerg Med* 1994;1:9–16.

23. Wolfson D, Lindberg E, Su L, et al. Three rapid immunoassays for the determination of creatine kinase MB: an analytical, clinical, and interpretive evaluation. *Amm Heart J* 1991;122:958–964.

24. Hedges JR, Young GP, Henkel GF, et al. Serial ECGs are less accurate than serial CK-MB results for emergency department diagnosis of myocardial infarction. *Ann Emerg Med* 1992;21: 1445–1450.

Other Biochemical Tests

12

SUMMARY OF TECHNOLOGY

Several serum markers are being evaluated for the diagnosis of AMI (1–3). The characteristics of an ideal marker include its presence in high concentration in myocardium and not in other tissues, its rapid and complete release after myocardial injury and in proportion to extent of injury, and its persistence in plasma for several hours to provide a convenient diagnostic window but not so long as to prevent detection of recurrent myocardial necrosis. Although there is probably no ideal marker available at present, several markers used in combination may be helpful for triage in the ED.

Myoglobin

Myoglobin is a heme protein that is present in all muscle tissue in a single form. Although it is ubiquitous, many characteristics of myoglobin suggest that it is a potentially powerful tool in the diagnosis of AMI and reperfusion. Thus myoglobin is a sensitive but not specific marker of AMI and requires exclusion of skeletal muscle injury. It is detectable soon after the onset of AMI (2 hours) and peaks at approximately 3 to 15 hours (4–7), and it can show a "staccato" pattern of release in the setting of AMI. Increased levels of myoglobin have been reported in patients with UAP, possibly indicating subclinical myocyte death or release of myoglobin from ischemic skeletal muscle in critically ill patients (8). Immunoassays are available for detection of myoglobin, both on a qualitative and quantitative basis.

Proteins of the Troponin Complex

The troponin complex is located on the thin filament on the contractile apparatus. It has three subunits—troponin-T (TnT; the tropomyosin-binding subunit), troponin-I (TnI; the actomyosin-adenosine triphosphate-inhibiting subunit), and troponin-C (TnC; the calcium-binding subunit) (2). The proteins of the regulatory troponin complex are expressed as isoforms in cardiac and skeletal muscle (9,10). These isoforms are the result of transcription of genes specific for the respective muscle type. TnC is not useful for diagnosis of AMI because cardiac and slow skeletal muscle troponin-C reveals identical amino acid compositions. In contrast, cardiac TnT and TnI (cTnT and cTnI) are encoded by different genes in cardiac muscle, slow skeletal muscle, and fast skeletal muscle. Highly specific antibodies to the cardiac isoforms of cTnT and cTnI have been developed and are undergoing investigation for use as screening tests for patients with acute coronary syndromes (11–15).

Cardiac Myosin Light Chains

The myosin molecule found both in cardiac and skeletal muscle consists of two heavy chains and two light chains that are discriminated on the basis of distinctive chemical and functional features. A variety of immunologic assays have been developed to detect human cardiac myosin light chains (CMLCs). Initial immunoassays encountered difficulties because of the use of polyclonal antibodies that produced cross-reactivity between cardiac and skeletal myosin light chains. Several investigators are attempting to develop monoclonal antibodies to recognize different epitopes on the myosin light chains to circumvent these diagnostic difficulties (3). Because CMLCs are continuously released after infarction (16), they may serve as a good serum marker to diagnose and quantify myocardial necrosis and AMI. They may also have a role in the identification of patients with UAP (8,17). Until reliable analytic methods are available, it is unclear whether CMLC determinations in the ED will offer significant clinical utility.

Carbonic Anhydrase III

Carbonic anhydrase III is an 18,000-Da cytoplasmic protein found in skeletal muscle but not in cardiac muscle. In patients with skeletal muscle damage, the ratio of myoglobin to carbonic anhydrase III remains constant, whereas in patients with AMI, the ratio shows a temporal pattern similar to that of myoglobin. This exciting diagnostic observation merits close monitoring because it may be extremely useful for triage in patients in the ED.

CRITIQUE
Scientific Basis

The various markers under clinical investigation have been proposed as diagnostic tools because of their release patterns after AMI and their relative specificities for differentiating AMI from skeletal muscle injury. Several studies have suggested that the determination of myoglobin and troponin may be useful in identifying patients with AMI who are at risk of serious cardiac events.

Myoglobin can be detected in more than two thirds of patients with AMI at 3 hours and in nearly all patients by 6 hours (4). However, it is increased in several other conditions besides AMI. A significant number of articles address the sensitivity and specificity of myoglobin for the diagnosis of AMI (1); most of these studies were not performed in the ED. One of the major problems with the data is an inconsistent definition of a positive test (4–8). The positivity criterion varies from 50 µg/mL to 150 µg/mL. Additionally, some articles used the mean as their cutoff point, and others used 2 SDs above the mean. Clearly the sensitivity and specificity of the test will vary with the criterion for test positivity. Another problem is that there were variable time periods after a patient's presentation to the CCU before testing was performed.

Troponin, a myocardial-specific protein, appears to be useful in identifying patients with both UAP and AMI (18–21) and in UAP may be of prognostic importance in identifying patients at risk for future cardiac events. The time of observed increase for cTnT and cTnI is about the same for CK-MB. The increase of the troponins persists for 4 to 7 days longer than CK-MB. When compared with CK-MB, late infarction detected by troponin will be considered a false-positive result, decreasing specificity. The early release of troponin is thought to occur from the cytoplasmic pool. The persistent increase comes from continued degradation of the protein bound pool (18–20). The troponins are now approved for routine diagnostic use.

All the studies evaluating cTnT are of patients admitted to the CCU. No studies evaluated patients presenting with symptoms of chest pain to the ED. In general, the patient populations being tested in those studies are not well described. Most articles present data in consecutive patients, but none describes the populations from which these patients came and the thresholds or decision practices at individual sites. Therefore there is variability in the prevalence of AMI in these populations. This raises the possibility of spectrum bias altering the sensitivities and specificities in some of the studies.

When defining sensitivity and specificity for cTnT, there is variability in the cutoff used to characterize the test. This makes direct comparisons difficult. Two articles addressed the value of cTnT in predicting prognosis. Both suggest that cTnT may offer some prognostic importance. Data also suggest that the sensitivity and specificity of the test are dependent on the time it is performed after a patient's presentation to the ED or admission to the CCU. Sensitivity may be as high as 100% at 10 to 120 hours and lower earlier and later in the patient's presentation.

Clinical Practicality

Serum determinations of myoglobin and cTnT can be performed using automated equipment in most hospitals throughout the United States. However, random access of samples is not possible for cTnT, and few clinical laboratories are staffed to provide 24-hour testing. The development of hand-held cassettes for the qualitative detection of serum markers is also occurring rapidly.

Data from Prospective Clinical Trials in the ED Setting

Studies of Test Sensitivity and Specificity: Many trials are ongoing at the present time. Several have been presented only in abstract form. The field is further complicated by the development by different manufacturers of immunoassays for the various serum markers and the lack of direct comparison between the various assay kits.

Johnson et al (22) studied 316 patients presenting to the ED with chest pain and measured serial cTnT levels. Published results are detailed in Table 12-1.

In another study comparing the sensitivities of four marker proteins for diagnosis of AMI in 25 patients presenting to the ED within 4 hours (median, 2.13 hours), blood samples were drawn every hour for the first 10 hours (10). The first increased cTnT level was seen in 50% of AMI patients within 4 hours, compared with only 25% for CK and CK-MB in the same time frame. However, the overall efficiency of making the diagnosis of AMI is not greater with cTnT compared with CK-MB.

Katus et al (23) have demonstrated the potential utility of an immunochemical cTnT test in patients with AMI. Diagnostic accu-

Table 12-1　Serial cTnT Levels in Patients with Chest Pain

Value	AMI	UAP	Nonischemic Chest Pain
Mean maximum cTnT in first 24 hours	3.2 ± 5.3	0.09 ± 0.21	0.03 ± 0.14
Patients with elevated maximum cTnT (%)	100	21	5

racy, correct identification of AMI with positive cTnT levels and non-AMI with negative cTnT levels, was 98% for cTnT vs 97% for CK-MB and remained at 98% until 5.5 days after ED presentation. cTnT was also increased in 37 of 79 patients with UAP (56%). Increases of serum cTnT were positively correlated with reversible ST-segment or T-wave changes on ECG, as well as with complications. Thus an increased cTnT in patients with UAP appears to be a harbinger of complications. The cTnT test was particularly useful in patients with skeletal muscle injury and suspected AMI, with an accuracy of 89% compared with 63% for CK-MB.

cTnI has also been found by Adams et al (9) to be a specific indicator of AMI while not being detected in patients with acute skeletal muscle injury, chronic skeletal muscle disease, or chronic kidney failure or in marathon runners. The release profile of cTnI is similar to that of cTnT; it appears, therefore, that the benefits of cTnT discussed above will also be seen with cTnI. Both of these serum markers for myocardial necrosis could possibly replace CK-MB as the marker of choice for AMI detection in the ED.

Antman et al (24) recently studied 100 patients admitted for evaluation of chest pain. The performance of a handheld rapid assay for qualitative detection of cTnT at the bedside was evaluated. The reference standard was at least one of World Health Organization (WHO) criteria, intranormal increase of total CK with increased CK-MB and a temporal pattern consistent with AMI, or histologic evidence of AMI at autopsy. Results are shown in Table 12-2.

A problem arises in the interpretation of the meaning of increased cTnT levels in patients with the clinical diagnosis of UAP. Hamm et al (25) found that cTnT was increased in 33 of 84 patients with UAP (39%), whereas only 3 patients had increased CK by immunoinhibition, not mass assay. Ten of the 33 with increased cTnT later had AMI in the hospital, and 5 of the 10 patients died. Only 1 of 51 patients with a negative serum cTnT serum test result had AMI ($P < 0.001$). It is not clear whether

Table 12-2   Performance of a Hand-Held Rapid Assay for cTnT

Hours Since Chest Pain	Sensitivity (%)	Specificity (%)
0–2	33	95
2–4	50	100
4–8	75	100
>8	86	86

small pockets of irreversible myocardial injury occur (and are detected by cTnT assays) in patients with UAP or whether cTnT is released from reversibly ischemic cells (26). The relatively long period of time (7 to 10 days) that troponin stays increased may actually indicate either unstable angina or an undiagnosed non–Q-wave AMI 5 days earlier. By the time of presentation, CK-MB has normalized.

Measurements of myoglobin obtained within 8 to 12 hours of the onset of infarction have sensitivities of greater than 95%, but a significant number of false-positive results can be seen from skeletal muscle injury and kidney failure (1). Several studies have shown that serial detection of myoglobin has increased sensitivity for AMI over CK (4–7,27). In one study (4) sensitivity improved from 62% on ED presentation to 100% 3 hours later, compared with 50% and 95%, respectively, for immunochemical CK-MB analyses.

Studies of the Clinical Impact of the Tests' Actual Use: There are no randomized controlled or even high-quality observation studies showing that the "stat" availability of any of these markers changes health care delivery, improves outcome, or leads to better quality care.

Data from Other Clinical Studies

In a study of hospitalized patients with chest pain, Ravkilde et al (28) found that the probability of death or serious cardiac events at 6 months was significantly lower in the 83 patients with a negative cTnT test compared with the 43 with a positive cTnT test.

Adams (29) studied 96 patients undergoing vascular surgery and 12 undergoing spinal surgery. Of the eight patients who sustained a perioperative AMI (diagnosed by a new wall-motion abnormality on echocardiogram), all had abnormally increased cTnI levels, whereas only six had increased CK-MB levels.

Generalizability to Different Settings

Generalizability is poor as a result of the lack of studies in the ED population and the noncomparability of studies resulting from different positive criterion choices. Because most studies are reported in single cutoff rather than ROC format, comparisons are difficult. This is especially important in that no studies address the ED population of patients who present with chest pain. Settings include diagnosis of AMI, coronary bypass grafting, and admission to the CCU and hospital. Populations studied are sometimes unclear; however, relatively standard definitions are used for diagnosis of AMI.

Applicability to Population Subgroups, Including Women and Minorities

There are insufficient data on women and minorities.

Cost Considerations

Earlier diagnosis of ruled-out AMI would permit earlier triage to either discharge or shortened length of stay. Until the tests are shown to be useful in improving physician decisionmaking (triage and treatment), it is difficult to justify their routine application in the ED. Although several chest pain centers utilize these techniques to help triage patients to "holding areas," there are currently only limited data from a few centers showing the cost-effectiveness of this approach. "Stat" testing increases the cost both in terms of reagents (extra tests), as well as necessary staff to perform the tests; however, this may be counterbalanced by fewer admissions of patients not requiring hospitalization and more expeditious treatment of patients with ACI.

Overall cost implications are uncertain at present. These tests are likely to be cost-effective if there is any improvement on the margin (eg, more costs avoided than incurred as a result of the adoption of the test). They may be very costly if no marginal benefit exists.

Special Concerns

Biochemical markers are most useful in the ED for those patients with persistently nondiagnostic ECGs. Studies reported in the literature frequently present data on a mixture of patients, some with diagnostic ECGs at presentation and others with nondiagnostic tracings. Assays for biochemical markers of myocardial necrosis must be interpreted in the context of the time-dependent process of

131

AMI. The diagnostic efficiency of a single specimen at a given point in time will vary depending on the specific marker and the number of hours elapsed since the onset of chest pain. Different results may be reported for the same marker depending on whether investigators used only a single specimen or evaluated serial specimens obtained at regular intervals after initial presentation. In addition, some markers may be more efficient at detecting AMI in patients who present early (eg, myoglobin), whereas others are useful for detecting patients who present late (eg. cTnT and cTnI).

Significant problems exist with unfamiliarity with new markers on the part of many primary care physicians that could lead to misinterpretation of laboratory results.

Of special concern is that it is unclear whether the evaluations of cTnT were done with blinding to either the reference standard or the test. However, most often the studies present a consecutive group of patients and perform statistical models on the data from these patients. Therefore blinding may not be applicable. There is uncertainty about whether cTnT is increased in conditions other than myocardial necrosis. In further studies of cTnT, there needs to be a clear definition of the blinding of the test and the reference standard and a better definition of the populations at risk. The study should be done on an ED population.

Other than new prospective studies, there may be enough data to do a metaanalysis of the ROC curve for cTnT, which should take into account the time after presentation to the ED. Although ROC curve analysis is the only adequate methodology for evaluating these biochemical markers, few articles present ROC curves. In those that do, data are not always presented in sufficient detail to allow a reexamination of the results. The methodology for finding the incremental value of cTnT could be a logistic-regression model. If serologic tests for AMI are conditionally dependent, it may not be adequate to examine them in a univariate analysis.

For myoglobin, both the highly time-dependent nature of this laboratory test and the possibility that the patient populations being examined are not adequate to generalize to patients in the ED are of major concern. Most of the data at the time of the working group's deliberations are reflective of patients admitted to the CCU, not those who present to the ED.

Both further prospective testing and metaanalysis of myoglobin should be done. Again, a clear definition of the test reference standard is necessary. ROC curve analysis is the only appropriate analysis for this technology, and this should be constructed using time after presentation as an independent variable. As with the troponin markers, the added value of myoglobin may be best studied using logistic regression models. A study is needed in which consecutive patients presenting to the ED get all available diagnostic tests. Patients should be followed through their hospital stay or after their discharge home from the ED. Without a multiple markers study, there will not be enough evidence to recommend one technology over another or to understand each test's incremental value.

A major difficulty in interpreting the results of clinical trials with biochemical markers is the lack of a clear gold standard. The WHO criteria are inadequate for many cases of AMI, especially when CK and CK-MB values are only minimally increased above the normal range. Some of the newer markers (eg, cTnT) may be more sensitive than the gold standard (CK-MB), leading to a mistaken impression of reduced specificity for AMI.

Primary Advantages

The new immunoassays for various serum markers, particularly the rapid bedside qualitative assay systems, are extremely attractive for ED triage because of the rapid turnaround time (usually less than 20 minutes), noninvasive nature of the test, lack of need for skilled laboratory personnel, and opportunity for serial testing during the period of evaluation in the ED (point-of-care triage). Currently, five times as many patients are admitted to the hospital with chest pain as those who have AMI. A more accurate test to assist appropriate triage could possibly improve cost-effectiveness of ED patients with chest pain.

cTnT may be as sensitive for AMI but less specific than CK-MB increase, possibly because cTnT detects minimal myocardial damage. Increase occurs at about the same time after AMI but lasts longer. Therefore cTnT may be more accurate. However, the data suggest no statistically significant difference in the ROC curves for cTnT and CK, and they are not known to be significantly different.

Myoglobin may be advantageous in the early diagnosis of AMI. However, myoglobin's sensitivity in early diagnosis at zero hour may not give an adequate negative predictive value, and so the test would need to be repeated for patients presenting very early.

Primary Disadvantages

First, there is a lack of extensive comparative studies of assay kits for the same marker by different manufacturers. Thus, although cTnT, cTnI, myoglobin, and CK-MB are all useful in diagnosing AMI, it is unclear which test (or tests) is superior. Second, because the ED triage of patients with chest pain syndromes will probably require more than one serum marker, the lack of a large number of studies that simultaneously measure more than one serum marker makes it difficult to determine which pattern of markers is most useful in the ED.

Increase of serum markers is not 100% sensitive for myocardial cell necrosis. An understanding of release kinetics for the various cardiac serum markers is necessary to obtain maximum clinical benefit for their use, particularly in the emergency setting. Early presentation of patients to the ED may provide false-negative results with all serum markers. Care also must be taken by the clinician not be release a patient from the ED on the basis of a negative serum marker series because ACI may be present without actual cellular necrosis.

Few randomized trials are available showing the effectiveness of these tests, both for the initial triage of patients in chest pain centers and EDs and holding areas, as well as in the use of thrombolytic therapy. There is a limited scientific basis for use, and there has been a poor description of the test results.

SUMMARY AND RECOMMENDATIONS

Myoglobin, an early marker of AMI, and cTnT and cTnI, which are specific for myocyte damage and are late markers, hold promise to improve the identification of patients with AMI and minor myocardial injury. However, the use of new biochemical markers in the ED as a routine measure to improve either the initial triage or therapy of patients with AMI is currently unproven. Although this information may be useful in those hospitals attempting to triage patients between ED holding areas and inpatient beds, the value of their approach needs further bolstering by additional data from carefully controlled studies.

Ultimately, serum protein testing may likely include a panel of multiple makers, which provide a spectrum of information regarding the time of AMI onset. An early sensitive marker such as myoglobin, when combined with CK-MB and cTnT (increased in the presence of AMI), could provide the clinician with critical

Table 12-3 Other Biochemical Tests

| | ED Diagnostic Performance | | ED Clinical Impact | |
	Quality of Evidence	Accuracy	Quality of Evidence	Impact
Troponin-T and troponin-1	B	For AMI: + + For UAP: NE	NK	NK
Myoglobin	B	For AMI: + For UAP: NE	NK	NK

information necessary to make decisions in the emergency setting.

Because thrombolytic therapy and primary angioplasty for AMI have been proved beneficial up to 12 hours after symptom onset, serum marker testing should become a mainstay in the diagnosis of AMI in the ED for patients with nondiagnostic ECGs or in age-undetermined left bundle-branch block. Such serum protein testing, if positive, could increase the clinician's use of electrocardiographic testing to indicate the potential evolution of ST-segment elevation in the patient with an initially nondiagnostic ECG and identify individuals with high likelihood for ischemic complications. Studies of biochemical serum markers of myocardial necrosis other than CK-MB in the ED setting are both appropriate and necessary for defining patterns of optimal care.

The results of the Working Group's final ratings of the quality of evidence evaluating these technologies and of their ED diagnostic performance and clinical impact are summarized in Table 12-3.

REFERENCES

1. Vaidga HC. Myoglobin. *Lab Med* 1992;23:306–310.
2. Katus HA, Scheffold T, Remppis A, et al. Proteins of the troponin complex. *Lab Med* 1992;23:311–317.
3. Weeds AG, Pope B. Chemical studies on light chains from cardiac and skeletal muscle myosin. *Nature* 1971;234:85–88.
4. Gibler WB, Gibler CD, Weinshenker E, et al. Myoglobin as an early indicator of acute myocardial infarction. *Ann Emerg Med* 1987;16:851–856.
5. Brogan GX, Friedman S, McCluskey C, et al. Evaluation of a new rapid quantitative immunoassay for serum myoglobin

versus CK-MB for ruling out acute myocardial infarction in the emergency department. *Ann Emerg Med* 1994;24:665–671.

6. Bakker AJ, Koelemay MJ, Gorgels JP, et al. Troponin-T and myoglobin at admission: value of early diagnosis of acute myocardial infarction. *Eur Heart J* 1994;15:45–53.

7. Ohman EM, Casey C, Bengtson JR, et al. Early detection of acute myocardial infarction: additional diagnostic information from serum concentrations of myoglobin in patients without ST elevation. *Br Heart J* 1990;63:335–338.

8. Hoberg E, Katus HA, Diederich KW, et al. Myoglobin, creatine kinase-B isoenzyme, and myosin light chain release in patients with unstable angina pectoris. *Eur Heart J* 1987;8:989–994.

9. Adams JE, Bodor GS, Davila-Roman VG, et al. Cardiac troponin I: a marker with high specificity for cardiac injury. *Circulation* 1993;88:101–106.

10. Mair J, Dienstl E, Puschendorf B. Cardiac troponin T in the diagnosis of myocardial injury. *Crit Rev Clin Lab Sci* 1992;29:31–57.

11. Bodor GS, Porter S, Landt Y, et al. Development of monoclonal antibodies for an assay of cardiac troponin-I and preliminary results in suspected cases of myocardial infarction. *Clin Chem* 1992;38:2203–2214.

12. Katus HA, Schoeppenthau M, Tanzeem A, et al. Non-invasive assessment of perioperative myocardial cell damage by circulating cardiac troponin-T. *Br Heart J* 1991;65:259–264.

13. Katus HA, Looser S, Hallermayer K, et al. Development and in vitro characterization of a new immunoassay of cardiac troponin-T. *Clin Chem* 1992;38:386–393.

14. Katus HA, Remppis A, Looser S, et al. Enzyme linked immunoassay of cardiac tropoinin-T for the detection of acute myocardial infarction in patients. *J Mol Cell Cardiol* 1989;21:1349–1353.

15. Larue C, Calzolari C, Bertinchant J-P, et al. Cardiac-specific immunoenzymometric assay of troponin I in the early phase of acute myocardial infarction. *Clin Chem* 1993;39:972–979.

16. Katus HA, Diedrich KW, Schwartz F, et al. Influence of reperfusion on serum concentrations of cytosolic creatine kinase and structural myosin light chains in acute myocardial infarction. *Am J Cardiol* 1987;60:440–445.

17. Katus HA, Diedrich KW, Hoberg E, et al. Circulating cardiac myosin light chains in patients with angina at rest: identification of a high risk subgroup. *J Am Coll Cardiol* 1988;11:487–493.

18. Gerhardt W, Katua HA, Rarkilde J, et al. S-troponin-T in suspected ischemic myocardial injury compared with mass and catalytic concentrations of s-creatine kinase isoenzyme MB. *Clin Chem* 1991;37:1405–1411.

19. Adams JE III, Schechtman KB, Landt Y, et al. Comparable detection of acute myocardial infarction by creatine kinase MB isoenzyme and cardiac toponin I. *Clin Chem* 1994;40:1291–1295.

20. Bakker AJ, Gorgels JP, van Vlies B, et al. The mass concentrations of serum troponin T and creatine kinase-MB are elevated before creatine kinase and creatine kinase-MB activities in acute myocardial infarction. *Eur J Clin Chem Biochem* 1993;31:715–724.

21. Mair J, Artner-Dworzak E, Lechleitner P, et al. Cardiac troponin-T in diagnosis of acute myocardial infarction. *Clin Chem* 1991;37:845–852.

22. Johnson PA, Albano MP, Sack D, et al. Troponin T in patients with acute chest pain (abstract). *J Am Coll Cardiol* 1994;23(1A):412A.

23. Katus HA, Remppis A, Nuemann FJ, et al. Diagnostic efficiency of troponin-T measurements in acute myocardial infarction. *Circulation* 1991;83:902–912.

24. Antman EM, Grudzien C, Sacks DB. Evaluation of a rapid bedside assay for the detection of cardiac troponin-T. *JAMA* 1995;273:1279–1282.

25. Hamm CW, Ravkilde J, Gerhardt W, et al. The prognostic value of serum troponin-T in unstable angina. *N Engl J Med* 1992;327:146–150.

26. Ellis AK. Serum protein measurements and the diagnosis of acute myocardial infarction. *Circulation* 1991;83:1107–1109.

27. Lee HS, Cross SJ, Garthwaite P, et al. Comparison of the value of novel rapid measurement of myoglobin, creatine kinase, and creatine kinase MB with the electrocardiogram for the diagnosis of acute myocardial infarction. *Br Heart J* 1994;71:311–315.

28. Ravkilde J, Horder M, Gerhardt W, et al. Diagnostic performance and prognostic value of serum troponin-T in suspected

acute myocardial infarction. *Scand J Clin Lab Invest* 1993;53:
677–685.

29. Adams JE III, Sicard GA, Allen BT, et al. Diagnosis of perioperative myocardial infarction with measurement of cardiac troponin 1. *N Engl J Med* 1994;330(10):670–674.

Echocardiogram

13

SUMMARY OF TECHNOLOGY

Echocardiography provides real-time two-dimensional images of the beating heart, and Doppler echocardiography provides real-time information about blood flow velocities in the heart. The echocardiogram is obtained with a transducer placed on the chest wall that both sends and receives ultrasound. After passing through the chest wall, the sound waves are reflected back to the transducer from the various interfaces that are encountered. The returning echo signals are converted into electrical energy, and the signals are amplified, processed, and displayed on an oscilloscope and recorded on videotape. The resulting images are readily recognizable moving displays of the pericardium, the myocardial walls, the cardiac chambers, the valves, and (with Doppler) the blood flow.

For the purposes of this analysis, the most important information concerns the visualization of the ventricular walls and endocardial surfaces. Images of the motion of all left ventricular segments are obtainable (interventricular septum, apex, posterior, anterior, lateral, and inferior walls); these may be further subdivided into subsegments for analysis, if necessary. In addition to wall motion, the degree of normal thickening of a myocardial segment (or lack thereof, with ischemia) may be assessed. In addition to an assessment of segmental wall motion and thickening, an estimation or measurement of global function (ejection fraction) is readily obtainable. To assist with triage, other patients who present with chest pain (such as pericarditis and aortic dissection) may be assessed with echocardiography. In addition, the patency of an internal mammary coronary artery bypass graft can be determined with Doppler techniques, which may be useful in evaluating post-CABG (coronary artery bypass graft) patients with chest pain. In addition, edge-detection ("acoustic quantification") is a newer technique that may aid in wall-motion analysis and global functional assessment (ejection fraction).

Although beyond the scope of this review, additional information is easily obtained about complications of infarction such as thrombus formation, septal rupture, papillary muscle rupture, mitral or tricuspid regurgitation without papillary muscle rupture, cardiac rupture, and pseudoaneurysm formation. In addition, mortality may be predictable with echocardiographic algorithms.

CRITIQUE
Scientific Basis

When myocardium becomes ischemic, there is a nearly immediate alteration in wall motion and the wall becomes hypokinetic or dyskinetic. This was documented in the 1970s in studies done on experimental infarction in animals, as well as in the 1980s with echocardiography performed during balloon inflation in coronary arteries in patients undergoing percutaneous transluminal coronary artery (PTCA) angioplasty (1). One limitation to the use of wall motion alone as an index of ischemia is that the movement of a myocardial segment is influenced by the motion of the adjacent segments; for example, if one segment is dyskinetic, adjacent nonischemic segments may be hypokinetic; conversely, if there is a hyperkinetic nonischemic segment, it may pull on an adjacent ischemic segment and make it move in a normal fashion. One way to avoid this pitfall is to evaluate systolic thickening of the myocardial wall as well as wall motion. A reduction is systolic thickening is a specific finding for myocardial ischemia. During acute ischemia or infarction, not only may the muscle fail to thicken, it may become thinner than normal, a very specific finding (a thinner wall during systole than during diastole). However, the echocardiogram cannot distinguish between ischemia and acute infarction. In addition, false-positive changes in wall motion may occur in patients with conduction abnormalities or right ventricular volume overload and after heart surgery.

These general findings have been used for localization of the specific coronary obstruction by echocardiography: When a wall motion abnormality is seen on echocardiography, there is a good chance of predicting which coronary artery is obstructed and causing the abnormality. This has been shown by correlating coronary angiography with exercise echocardiography and also by correlating echocardiography with angiography in patients having an acute myocardial infarction (AMI). For example, on the long axis echocardiographic view, the interventricular septum as visualized is perfused by the left anterior descending (LAD) coronary artery, and the basal 1 to 2 cm of the septum is perfused by the part of the LAD proximal to the first septal perforator artery. The posterior wall as seen on the long axis view is perfused by the circumflex artery (and is therefore usually moving normally in the typical patient with inferior infarction). On the short axis view, the anterior free wall and the anterior septum are supplied by the LAD, the posteromedial free wall and the posterior septum are supplied by the posterior descending coronary artery, and the posterolateral wall is supplied by the circumflex. On the apical two-chamber view, the anterior wall is supplied by the LAD and the inferior wall by the posterior descending branch of the right coronary artery (RCA). On the apical four-chamber view, the apex and distal two thirds of the septum are LAD territory, the proximal septum is supplied by the posterior descending artery, and the lateral wall is supplied by the circumflex.

A key issue is the specific detection of AMI. Dramatic changes have been noted with the use of m-mode echocardiography 1 hour after the production of experimental AMI produced by the injection of microspheres into the circumflex coronary artery in dogs. In this experiment, both global and regional function decreased: stroke volume index decreased 49%, fractional shortening decreased 52%, lateral wall motion decreased 80%, lateral wall thickening decreased 100%, and end-systolic diameter increased 36% (all within 1 hour of infarction). (Studies at 6 days showed that wall motion had improved, but thickening did not return.)

In human patients, echocardiography has been compared with magnetic resonance imaging (MRI) (2) and with contrast angiography after AMI (3). In the former study (2), 17 patients underwent both MRI and two-dimensional echocardiography for the evaluation of segmental wall motion after AMI; however, only 11 were evaluated during the "acute" phase (up to 2 weeks after AMI in this study). One patient was excluded for a poor-quality MRI and one for a poor-quality echocardiogram. For comparison, seven patients also had contrast angiography and five had radionuclide angiography. Eleven segments were evaluated with both techniques with a scoring system. Both echocardiography and MRI detected wall-motion abnormalities in the LAD distribution; however, only echocardiography reliably detected abnormalities in the RCA distribution. There was significant interobserver agreement with both techniques. In the latter study (3), echocardiography and contrast angiography were compared in 20 patients within 12 hours of the onset of chest pain due to AMI. Anterior infarction was present in 10 and inferior in 10. Sixteen segments were evaluated with echocardiography, using a scoring system. In this study, echocardiography and angiography yielded similar results; however, the correlation between the two derived indexes of wall motion was lower than the authors expected. They explained this by noting that the angiographic index was derived based on SDs from normal ventriculograms, whereas the echocardiographic index was based on actual scores from abnormal wall motion. Second, the angiographic index reflected hyperkinesis in the noninfarct regions and the echocardiographic index did not. Third, when limited to the right anterior oblique view, the angiogram did not visualize the septum and posterior wall, whereas the echocardiogram visualized these areas well.

From these direct studies, it has been shown that echocardiography can promptly and accurately detect wall–motion and wall–thickening changes that occur during acute ischemia and infarction, which, along with its ability to detect other cardiac abnormalities, has created significant interest in its ED use for detection of ACI and AMI. However, few studies of the type described above were performed in the ED setting, and the primary issue is whether these findings have diagnostic and practical utility in the ED.

Clinical Practicality

It is necessary for an experienced sonographer or physician to perform adequate studies to assess wall motion (4,5). This requires five to six views (parasternal long-axis and short-axis views; apical four-chamber, two-chamber, and long-axis views; and subcostal views if necessary). Studies that concentrate on wall motion to minimize the amount of time for a patient in pain typically can be accomplished in 10 to 15 minutes. An acceptable imaging machine is mandatory, as is immediate sonographer availability. The study is accessible and noninvasive and can be performed at the bedside. Inadequate studies occur in approximately 10% of patients as a result of poor acoustic windows and patient uncooperativeness. After the performance of the examination, the study must be interpreted by experienced overreaders.

In the ED clinical context, it must be well appreciated that the acquisition of echocardiographic images is far more difficult than the recording of an ECG, and the skills necessary to interpret the recorded images are more difficult to acquire than those necessary to interpret an ECG. The acquisition of echocardiographic images is extremely operator dependent. Although more than 90% of patients have echocardiograms that are technically satisfactory for interpretation, this is only true when expert technicians are acquiring the images. Less well-trained technicians will produce a much lower yield of interpretable images, no matter how long they have been practicing their profession. In addition, no matter how excellent the training, people who have not had a long experience acquiring these images (eg, cardiology fellows) will also have a lower yield of interpretable images.

Further, the analysis of wall motion and myocardial thickening is one of the most challenging aspects of echocardiogram interpretation. Although published small series show a small interobserver variability, in the day-to-day function of the echocardiography laboratory, it is not unusual for one cardiologist who is an expert echocardiographer to ask for a second opinion regarding wall motion or thickening. In addition, the various systems of wall motion analysis involve a complex interpretation of multiple segments in at least four echocardiographic views.

Thus, although echocardiograms are rapidly obtainable and can be rapidly interpreted, both of these functions require personnel with specialized training and experience. During normal working hours, these skills are readily and rapidly available because expert echocardiography technicians can easily go immediately to the ED and the studies can be immediately interpreted by expert echocardiographers. However, at night there would be substantial delays in both of these processes. Practically speaking, ED personnel could also rapidly obtain the images and interpret them; however, as opposed to the more easily recognized entities such as pericardial effusion, the evaluation of wall motion and thickening by these personnel is unlikely to yield satisfactory accuracy.

Data from Prospective Clinical Trials in the ED Setting

Studies of Test Sensitivity and Specificity: Sasaki et al (6) performed echocardiography on 46 ED patients who were admitted for chest discomfort with normal ECGs and creatinine kinase. They excluded patients with prior AMI, significant valvular heart disease, cardiomyopathy, prior cardiac surgery, and left bundle-branch block.

Eight of 18 patients undergoing echocardiography during chest pain had wall-motion abnormalities. Six of the eight patients with positive echocardiography findings had AMIs. One of the 10 patients without wall-motion abnormalities had an AMI. Of the 28 patients who had echocardiography performed after relief of chest pain, 10 had abnormal studies and 18 had normal studies. Eight of 10 patients with abnormal studies had AMIs, and none of the 18 patients with normal studies had AMIs. *During chest pain*, sensitivity of echocardiography for detecting infarct was 86% and specificity was 82%. In the *absence of ongoing chest pain*, sensitivity was 100% and specificity was 90% in this small sample. As a preliminary study, from these results one may conclude the following: 1) a positive study finding during pain or after the pain had stopped correlated with the development of AMI or significant CAD, 2) a negative study finding after the pain had stopped did not detect underlying CAD in a significant percentage, and 3) a negative study during pain does not eliminate the possibility of AMI.

Peels et al (7) studied 43 patients with nondiagnostic ECGs in the ED. Again, patients without prior AMI, with known CAD, or who had procedures were excluded from the study, as were patients whose echo window was technically inadequate. Imaging was done *before relief of chest pain*, as soon as possible. Sensitivity for ACI was 88% (22 of 25) with a specificity of 78% (14 of 18). Sensitivity for AMI was 92% (12 of 13) with a specificity of 53% (16 of 30). Regional asynergy could not distinguish ischemia from infarction. The incidence of one-, two-, and three-vessel CAD was similar. The three patients without regional asynergy during pain but with coronary disease had single-vessel disease. The 17 patients with regional asynergy during pain had multivessel disease. Those patients with multivessel disease had more regional involvement than those with single-vessel disease in the 13 wall-segment models. Although these results are somewhat encouraging, aside from the very small size of this study, the fraction of ED patients to which its results are applicable is questionable; namely, only those without technical limitations or precluding history who are having ongoing chest pain.

Sabia et al (8) also evaluated regional wall-motion abnormalities prospectively in the ED. They studied 185 patients during 202 ED visits for chest pain or shortness of breath. These authors did not exclude patients with known prior coronary disease. Echocardiography was performed immediately, and the clinician was not made aware of the results. Standard views were used to evaluate 12 myocardial segments. Additional attention was paid to exclude complications of AMI, pericardial effusion, cardiac tamponade, and aortic dissection. The studies were read by three observers blinded to clinical status, ECG, and enzymes. They found a 94% technically adequate study rate. Of the 60 patients without regional or global dysfunction, 2 (4%) had AMIs. None of the 22 patients with global dysfunction without regional variation had an AMI. Of the 87 patients with regional wall motion, with or without global changes, 31% experienced AMIs. Nine of the 13 patients with AMI had normal ECGs, but all 13 had regional wall-motion abnormalities on two-dimensional echocardiography. If triage decisions had been made on the basis of echocardiogram results, it was projected that hospital stay would have been reduced by 23% and total charges would have been reduced by 24% (including the cost of the studies). No validation of these findings has been reported. Although this is the most encouraging study to date, the practicality of a three-observer rating and concerns about the remaining false-negative rate remain significant issues.

Studies of the Clinical Impact of the Test's Actual Use: No interventional clinical trials of the use of echocardiography for real-time decisionmaking for ED triage have yet been reported.

Data from Other Clinical Studies

Horowitz et al (9) initially performed two-dimensional echocardiography in 80 patients within 12 hours of admission to the CCU. Again, patients with preexisting reasons for left ventricular hypokinesis were excluded from the study. Thirty-one of 33 patients who had AMI had wall-motion abnormalities, and 27 of 32 patients without AMI had normal wall motion. The sensitivity for detecting infarction was 94% with a specificity of 84% in this CCU population. The ED population would be expected to have a lower prevalence of infarct than a CCU population, however, and the positive predictive value of echocardiography would be anticipated to be less. Moreover, 19% of patients had studies that were not acceptable for interpretation, including about half of those with AMI, and in the busy ED setting, imaging likely would be more difficult, resulting in even more uninterpretable results. In a recently published large retrospective study by Gibler et al (10), a negative echocardiogram strongly indicated no "cardiac disease," but positive studies were rare (19 of 901 studied patients) in this "heart ED" population, and of those, fewer than half (9) had any form of cardiac disease.

Oh et al (11) used echocardiography in four patients to direct management in the CCU. Detection of regional wall-motion abnormalities was used to guide reperfusion therapy; the clinical applicability of this approach deserves further study; its potential practical use in the ED is not clear.

Generalizability to Different Settings

Although the equipment is readily available (although expensive), a potential problem is that the accuracy of echocardiography is highly dependent on the quality of the images obtained, the skill of the operator, and the knowledge and experience of the interpreter. Therefore it is not clear that this technique will be widely applicable to the smaller community hospital or rural setting.

Applicability to Population Subgroups, Including Women and Minorities

Although there are no clear reasons to expect major problems in subgroups, there are no substantial data on which to judge the accuracy or reliability of echocardiography for detecting ACI in the ED setting in racial minorities, the elderly, and women. However, it is of note that in most studies, and presumably when applied to practice, more elderly people are disqualified for study because of their higher prevalence of CAD and prior AMI.

Cost Considerations

State-of-the-art echocardiography machines are costly (>$200,000) and need to be used frequently to justify this expense. The additional salaries for a 24-hour-a-day sonographer or the additional cost of training several ED physicians to perform these tests in a timely manner is significant (12). The interpretation of wall-motion abnormalities can be difficult, and ongoing review is necessary with overreading physicians. The potential savings discussed above projected as a result of improved triage have yet to be verified.

Special Concerns

The skills required to perform and interpret two-dimensional echocardiography are considerable. Minimal echocardiography training requirements for cardiologists include more than 3 months of an 80% effort into performing and/or interpreting more than 150 studies with direct supervision by the laboratory director (13). Additionally, there is a 10% inadequate-examination rate generally accepted in routine studies; this would likely be higher in patients in the ED who are in pain at the time of the examination. The likelihood of studying the patient during active chest pain is variable. Again, echocardiographic identification of wall-motion abnormalities cannot reliably distinguish acute infarct from ischemia or old infarct. Last, transmural ischemia is more likely to be evident with echocardiography than is subendocardial (nontransmural) disease.

On the basis of the approximately 8% false-negative rate from the prospective studies reviewed above, echocardiography cannot be used in isolation to reduce the utilization of medical resources by discharging all patients with negative studies. Also, this number occurred despite the fact that the studies were done as part of a planned investigation and the results were determined by a majority or consensus of experts.

Primary Advantages

Echocardiography is rapid, accessible, safe, and essentially painless and gives real-time information. An experienced overreader can interpret the study at the patient's bedside. Other unsuspected diagnoses can be identified, such as right heart disease (pulmonary embolism), valvular heart disease, aortic dissection, pericardial effusion/tamponade, and complications of AMI.

Primary Disadvantages

A dedicated experienced sonographer will optimize the quality of the results, and anything short of this will reduce any sensitivity/specificity data reported. Echocardiography is poor at distinguishing active from old ischemic events, and this clearly limits the usefulness of the test. Also, patients who present to the ED with a chest pain syndrome very often do not have it at the time of their presentation; we know from stress echocardiography data that wall-motion abnormalities can resolve within a minute of maximal stress.

At a practical level, as reviewed above, a number of problems are revealed in the currently available data: 1) the false-negative rates in the prospective studies are too high to be safe; 2) in particular, false positives may occur in patients with conduction changes, with right ventricular volume overload, and after heart surgery; 3) selection of the target population is not yet defined; 4) the approximate number of studies technically inadequate for interpretation is 10%; 5) studies must be done by expert technicians; 6) studies must be interpreted by expert echocardiographers, cardiologists subspecializing in echocardiography, who may not be available in smaller institutions; 7) studies do not always distinguish between new and old infarctions; and 8) the complex scoring systems used in the prospective studies may not be practical.

SUMMARY AND RECOMMENDATIONS

Although echocardiography in the ED showed initial promise, it is labor-intensive and insensitive for distinguishing new from old ischemia. Its use in the absence of chest pain appears to be more accurate in a single study with low numbers for unclear reasons. It can be recommended as an adjunctive test if readily available during atypical chest pain; there are insufficient data demonstrating that it can effectively triage patients in large clinical settings.

Echocardiography is a generally accurate technique, but in the ED setting when looking for ACI, it still has a false-negative rate that precludes discharging all patients with negative echocardiography findings. For the purpose of ruling in or ruling out AMI, echocardiography cannot be done accurately by ED personnel. During hours when expert technicians and interpreters are readily available, echocardiography might improve the accuracy of diagnosis and might thereby lead to a reduction in unnecessary admissions and costs. Beyond the diagnosis of ACI, for those with AMI, additional potentially useful clinical information about complications and hemodynamic status (ejection fraction, pulmonary artery pressure) would also become known, possibly leading to improvements in management and prognosis. Study results that suggest alternative diagnoses that need acute care would also be potentially beneficial.

However, overall, the available investigations to date suggest that even in a *selected* ED population, echocardiography may be reasonably specific but not clearly sufficiently sensitive for either ACI or AMI for this tool to be recommended for ED use. Its role for the overall ED population is even less clear and cannot be recommended without much more information about which patients for

Table 13-1 Echocardiogram

ED Diagnostic Performance		ED Clinical Impact	
Quality of Evidence	Accuracy	Quality of Evidence	Impact
B	+	NK	NK

whom it should be considered, its diagnostic performance in the usual ED setting, and its safety and effectiveness in this setting when tested in a controlled interventional clinical trial.

The results of the Working Group's final ratings of the quality of evidence evaluating this technology and of its ED diagnostic performance and clinical impact are given in Table 13-1.

REFERENCES

1. Hauser G, Gangadharan V, Ramos R, et al. Sequence of mechanical, electrocardiographic and clinical effects of repeated coronary occlusion in human beings: echocardiographic observations during coronary angioplasty. *J Am Coll Cardiol* 1985;5:193–197.
2. White RD, Cassidy MM, Sheitlin MD, et al. Segmental evaluation of left ventricular wall motion after myocardial infarction. Magnetic resonance imaging versus echocardiography. *Am Heart J* 1988;115:166–175.
3. Lundgren C, Bourdillon PD, Dillon JC, et al. Comparison of contrast angiography and two-dimensional echocardiography for the evaluation of left ventricular regional wall motion abnormalities after acute myocardial infarction. *Am J Cardiol* 1990;65:1071–1077.
4. Gardner CJ, Brown S, Hagen-Ansert S, et al. Guidelines for cardiac sonographer education: report of the American Society of Echocardiography Sonographer Education and Training Committee. *J Am Soc Echo* 1992;5:635–639.
5. Pearlman AS, Gardin JM, Martin RP, et al. Guidelines for optimal physician training in echocardiography. Recommendations of the American Society of Echocardiography Committee for Physician Training in Echocardiography. *Am J Cardiol* 1987;60:158–163.
6. Sasaki H, Charuzi Y, Beeder C, et al. Utility of echocardiography for the early assessment of patients with non-diagnostic chest pain. *Am Heart J* 1986;112:494–497.
7. Peels CH, Visser CA, Funke-Kupper AJ, et al. Usefulness of two-dimensional echocardiography for immediate detection of myocardial ischemia in the emergency room. *Am J Cardiol* 1990;65:687–691.
8. Sabia P, Afrookteh A, Touchstone DA, et al. Value of regional wall motion abnormality in the emergency room diagnosis of acute myocardial infarction: a prospective study using two-

dimensional echocardiography. *Circulation* 1991;84(suppl I): I85–I92.

9. Horowitz RS, Morganroth J, Parrotto C, et al. Immediate diagnosis of acute myocardial infarction by two-dimensional echocardiography. *Circulation* 1982:65:323–329.

10. Gibler WB, Runyon JP, Levy RC, et al. A rapid diagnostic and treatment center for patients with chest pain in the emergency department. *Ann Emerg Med* 1995;25:1–8.

11. Oh JK, Miller FA, Shub C, et al. Evaluation of acute chest pain syndromes by two-dimensional echocardiography: its potential application in the selection of patients for acute reperfusion therapy. *Mayo Clin Proc* 1987;62:59–66.

12. Hauser AM. The emerging role of echocardiography in the emergency department. *Ann Emerg Med* 1989;18:1298–1303.

13. DeMaria AN, Crawford MH, Feigenbaum H, et al. Task force IV: training in echocardiography. *J Am Coll Cardiol* 1986;7: 1207–1208.

Thallium Scanning

14

SUMMARY OF TECHNOLOGY

More than two decades of clinical experience in patients with known or suspected coronary artery disease indicate that thallium-201 is an excellent perfusion tracer that can be used to identify patients with ACI occurring spontaneously or provoked by exercise or pharmacologic stress (1–5). Thallium-201, injected intravenously, is taken up by the myocardium in proportion to regional coronary blood flow (6). The regional distribution of the tracer can then be imaged with the use of a standard Anger camera (gamma camera). Thallium-201 also washes out of the myocardium in proportion to blood flow, and subsequent images taken several hours after injection ("redistribution" images) can be used to determine whether the initial perfusion defect results from fibrotic or necrotic myocardium (in which case the defect is irreversible) or from ischemic myocardium (in which case the defect shows improvement or reversibility with time) (7).

Thallium scanning has been shown to be useful for predicting risk of recurrent AMI and death after admission for AMI (4,5,8–16). Evidence of reversible ischemia provoked by either exercise or pharmacologic testing is associated with worsened long-term outcome.

CRITIQUE
Scientific Basis

It has been well established in a large number of laboratory conditions that the regional myocardial uptake of thallium-201 is proportional to regional blood flow. In addition, the extraction of thallium, a cation, is analogous to that of potassium ion and requires active processes at the level of the sarcolemma. Hence thallium uptake is a marker of cell membrane integrity and, even if blood flow is restored, thallium is not retained in acutely or chronically infarcted myocardium. In contrast, retention of thallium with time, or even net increase in myocardial tracer activity with time, has been well demonstrated in experimental models of acute myocardial ischemia (7).

Thallium scanning as an excellent means of detecting myocardial necrosis, as well as reduced coronary blood flow and perfusion. Several studies have shown that the extent of AMI as measured by thallium scanning is related to both the resulting ejection fraction and long-term cardiac events (death, AMI, recurrent angina, need for revascularization) (4,5,17–19). Several clinical trials have demonstrated that reversible perfusion abnormalities in selected groups of patients before discharge after AMI are associated with an increased risk for recurrent infarction or mortality (8,9,11–16). However, there are no data at present to show that interventions in these groups of patients are effective at altering outcome. Numerous other studies have shown that thallium scanning is a very accurate imaging technique to identify patients with multi-vessel coronary disease (4,5,20–23). In addition, thallium imaging is useful for identifying viable myocardium that will improve in function after revascularization in patients with left ventricular dysfunction after AMI (24).

Clinical Practicality

Resting perfusion imaging with a portable gamma camera is practical in the ED setting. However, thallium requires a cyclotron for production and is usually produced in a few central facilities and shipped to hospital nuclear medicine laboratories on a daily basis. Thus the unavailability of the isotope after normal working hours may limit its practicality for this purpose. (In an institution that uses thallium-201 routinely this may not be a problem. Thallium-201 can be delivered to the ED every 2 to 3 days to ensure a steady supply.)

This aside, because of redistribution, to obtain a useful image in the context of diagnosing ACI/AMI, scanning should be done immediately after injection. This limits the usefulness of this technique for ED patients, as it is impractical to move a patient who has just presented with chest pain to the nuclear medicine department for imaging (5).

Data from Prospective Clinical Trials in the ED Setting

Numerous studies have documented the usefulness of thallium-201 scanning for the diagnosis of coronary disease (1–5), the diagnosis of infarction (17,25), and the evaluation of patients after thrombolysis (26–30) or revascularization procedures (31–37). Thallium imaging has also been applied to patients with ACI (38–42). However, for this review, of 81 articles found on literature search of the use of thallium-201 in AMI, only 3 pertained to its ED use; 2 were prospective and 1 retrospective, as reviewed below.

Studies of Test Sensitivity and Specificity: The one prospective study, by van der Wieken et al (43), included 149 patients at one institution with acute chest pain and nondiagnostic ECGs. The interval between pain and scanning was 12 hours or less. Defects were present in 57 patients: AMI developed in 35, infarction developed within 2 months in 7, 10 had the diagnosis of coronary disease made by angiography or stress-thallium-201 testing, and in 5 chest pain was of probable noncardiac origin. An equivocal scan was present in 13, and coronary disease was present or strongly suggested in 5. A normal scan was present in 79: 1 had AMI, stress testing was positive in 6, and stress testing was negative in 72. There were no cardiac events in these 72 patients during the subsequent year. The conclusion was that there was high sensitivity (97%) and relatively high specificity (77%).

Studies of the Clinical Impact of the Test's Actual Use: There are no studies of clinical impact.

Data from Other Clinical Studies

In a retrospective study by Hennemann et al (44), thallium-201 scans and technetium-99m first-pass angiography were evaluated in a convenience sample of 47 patients in the ED who presented with chest pain and nondiagnostic ECGs. AMI developed in only four patients, as diagnosed by CK-MB subunit 6% or greater of total CK. The combined scans had a sensitivity of 75% and a specificity of 42%. The positive predictive value was only 11%, but the negative predictive value was 95%. The authors concluded that the scans were not useful, but the number of infarctions was much too small to make any meaningful comparisons, and the study was retrospective.

Mace et al (45) conducted portable thallium-201 scans in 20 consecutive patients with chest pain; 12 had equivocal symptoms and ECGs, and 8 had classical presentations. A second scan was done 1 hour later if the initial one was abnormal. Infarction did develop in all three patients with scans indicative of infarction (all three had presented atypically). There were no infarctions among the 14 with negative scans. No follow-up was reported. Unfortunately, this study is too small to be meaningful.

Generalizability to Different Settings

Thallium imaging is widely available in most hospital settings, and the findings of the above reports should be reproducible in most centers. However, results will be dependent on the skill and experience of the interpreting physician. Difficulties associated with radionuclide handling by trained personnel and quality control of imaging make this a cumbersome and labor-intensive test to apply in the ED on a 24-hour basis.

Applicability to Population Subgroups, Including Women and Minorities

The principles of thallium imaging should apply well to both women and minorities. However, in women, artifacts caused by breast tissue frequently produce an apparent anterior defect, and in both sexes diaphragmatic artifacts may produce an apparent inferior defect.

Cost Considerations

Thallium imaging would increase the costs of the evaluation of the chest pain patient. Typical costs are in the range of $500 to $800. Thus such imaging should be considered only in selected patient subgroups. This is on the order of $150 less than the cost of a similar study with sestamibi.

Special Concerns

Special concerns include those issues listed below as disadvantages and the fact that almost no prospective data exist about the actual use of thallium imaging in the ED.

Primary Advantages

Thallium imaging is widely used, and most nuclear medicine physicians and nuclear cardiologists have extensive training in its use and interpretation. The imaging equipment (a portable gamma camera) is available in most institutions.

Primary Disadvantages

As with other radioisotopes, patients must be moved from the ED to be scanned. Also, thallium-201 is not an optimal isotope for clinical imaging with a gamma camera. Its low-energy photons are easily scattered and attenuated, and its half-life is 73 hours. Because of the radiation exposure resulting from the long half-life, the dose of thallium that is injected must be kept low (in the order of 2 to 4 mCi). This, in combination with the low energy of thallium-201, results in images that are poorer in quality than images that can be obtained with technetium-99m. Because thallium distribution in the myocardium is not static but changes with time, imaging must commence within 15 to 20 minutes after injection, which may be impractical in some patients with acute chest pain. Moreover, only experts in nuclear medicine can interpret the scans. This latter concern may be overcome by teleradiology, which is more easily done for nuclear scans than for typical radiographs. Additionally, the test's diagnostic performance in the ED setting is not known at this point and may not be sufficient to be helpful. Finally, the lack of isotope availability, noted above, will limit the practicality of thallium imaging for this purpose during other than normal working hours.

SUMMARY AND RECOMMENDATIONS

The use of resting radionuclide imaging for the diagnosis of ACI/AMI in the ED should be restricted to specialized and limited situations in which the clinical triad of history, ECG changes, and enzymatic/laboratory measurements is not available or is unreliable. Such imaging may be helpful, for example, in patients with equivocal chest pain histories and nondiagnostic ECG findings. Thallium-201 is an excellent perfusion tracer, but the available data indicate relatively poor diagnostic accuracy in the setting of AMI or unstable angina, with a particularly low specificity. There are also difficulties with isotope availability and tracer redistribution

Table 14-1 Thallium Scanning

ED Diagnostic Performance		ED Clinical Impact	
Quality of Evidence	Accuracy	Quality of Evidence	Impact
C	NK-NE	NK	NK-NE

(necessitating imaging with 15 to 20 minutes after injection). Hence thallium-201 does not appear to be an ideal agent for use in the ED management of patients with chest pain.

The results of the Working Group's final ratings of the quality of evidence evaluating this technology and of its ED diagnostic performance and clinical impact are detailed in Table 14-1.

REFERENCES

1. Verani MS, Marcus ML, Razzak MA, et al. Sensitivity and specificity of thallium-201 perfusion imaging under exercise in the diagnosis of coronary artery disease. *J Nucl Med* 1978;19: 773–782.
2. Maddahi J, Van Train K, Prigent F, et al. Quantitative single photon emission computed thallium-201 tomography for detection and localization of coronary artery optimization and prospective validation of a new technique. *J Am Coll Cardiol* 1989;14:1689–1699.
3. Zaret BL, Wackers FJ, Soufer R. Nuclear cardiology. In Braunwald E, ed. *Heart Disease: A Textbook of Cardiovascular Medicine.* 4th ed. Philadelphia: WB Saunders, 1992:276–311.
4. Zaret BL, Wackers FJ. Nuclear cardiology. *N Engl J Med* 1993; 329:775–783, 855–863.
5. Ritchie JL, Bateman TM, Bonow RO, et al. Guidelines for clinical use of cardiac radionuclide imaging. A report of the American Heart Association/American College of Cardiology Task Force on Assessment of Diagnostic and Therapeutic Cardiovascular Procedures. *Circulation* 1995;91:1278–1302.
6. Strauss HW, Harrison K, Langan JK, et al. Thallium-201 for myocardial imaging: relation of thallium-201 to regional myocardial perfusion. *Circulation* 1975;51:641–645.
7. Beller GA, Watson DD, Pohost GM. Kinetics of thallium distribution and redistribution: clinical applications in sequential myocardial imaging. In Strauss HW, Pitt B, eds. *Cardiovascular Nuclear Medicine.* 2nd ed. St. Louis: Mosby, 1979:225–242.
8. Gibson RS, Watson DD, Craddock GB, et al. Predication of cardiac events after uncomplicated myocardial infarction: a prospective study comparing predischarge exercise thallium-201 scintigraphy and coronary angiography. *Circulation* 1983; 68:321–333.
9. Hung J, Goris ML, Nash E, et al. Comparative value of maximal treadmill testing, exercise thallium myocardial perfu-

sion scintigraphy and exercise radionuclide ventriculography for distinguishing high- and low-risk patients perfusion scintigraphy and exercise radionuclide ventriculography for distinguishing high- and low-risk patients soon after acute myocardial infarction. *Am J Cardiol* 1984;53:1221–1227.

10. Beller GA, Gibson RS. Risk stratification after myocardial infarction. *Mod Concepts Cardiovasc Dis* 1986;55:5–10.

11. Brown KA, Weiss RM, Clements JP, et al. Usefulness of residual ischemic myocardium within prior infarct zone for identifying patients at high risk after acute myocardial infarction. *Am J Cardiol* 1987;60:15–19.

12. Leppo JA, O'Brien J, Rothendler JA, et al. Dipyridamole thallium-201 scintigraphy in the prediction of future cardiac events after myocardial infarction. *N Engl J Med* 1985;310:1014–1018.

13. Gibson RS, Beller GA, Gheorghiade M, et al. The prevalence and clinical significance of residual myocardial ischemia two weeks after uncomplicated non-Q-wave infarction: a prospective natural history study. *Circulation* 1986;73:1186–1198.

14. Younis LT, Byers S, Shaw L, et al. Prognostic value of intravenous dipyridamole-thallium scintigraphy after acute myocardial ischemic events. *Am J Cardiol* 1989;64:161–166.

15. Gimple LW, Hutter AM, Guiney TE, et al. Prognostic utility of predischarge dipyridamole thallium imaging compared to predischarge submaximal exercise electrocardiography and maximal exercise thallium imaging after uncomplicated acute myocardial infarction. *Am J Cardiol* 1989;64:1243–1248.

16. Brown KA, O'Meara J, Chambers CE, et al. Ability of dipyridamole thallium-201 imaging one to four days after acute myocardial infarction to predict in-hospital and late recurrent myocardial ischemic events. *Am J Cardiol* 1990;65:160–167.

17. Wackers FJ, Sokole EB, Samson G, et al. Value and limitations of thallium-201 scintigraphy in the acute phase of myocardial infarction. *N Engl J Med* 1976;295:1–5.

18. Hakki AH, Nestico PF, Heo J, et al. Relative prognostic value of rest thallium-201 imaging, radionuclide ventriculography and 24-hour ambulatory electrocardiographic monitoring after acute myocardial infarction. *J Am Coll Cardiol* 1987;10:25–32.

19. Cerqueira MD, Maynard C, Ritchie JL, et al. Long-term survival in 618 patients from the Western Washington Streptokinase in Myocardial Infarction trials. *J Am Coll Cardiol* 1992;20:1452–1459.

20. Nygaard TN, Griffith RS, Ryan JM, et al. Prevalence of high-

risk thallium-201 scintigraphic findings in left main coronary artery stenosis: comparison with patients with multiple- and single-vessel coronary artery disease. *Am J Cardiol* 1984;53: 462–469.

21. Maddahi J, Abdulla A, Garcia EV, et al. Noninvasive identification of left main and triple vessel coronary artery disease: improved accuracy using quantitative analysis of regional myocardial stress distribution and washout of thallium-201. *J Am Coll Cardiol* 1986;7:53–60.

22. Christian TF, Miller TD, Bailey KR, et al. Noninvasive identification of severe coronary artery disease using exercise tomographic thallium-201 imaging. *Am J Cardiol* 1992;70:14–20.

23. Iskandrian AS, Heo J, Lemiek J, et al. Identification of high-risk patients with left main and three-vessel coronary artery disease using stepwise discriminant analysis of clinical, exercise, and tomographic thallium data. *Am Heart J* 1993;125:221–225.

24. Dilsizian V, Bonow RO. Current diagnostic techniques of assessing myocardial viability in hibernating and stunned myocardium. *Circulation* 1993;87:1–20.

25. Wackers FJ, Becker AE, Samson G, et al. Location and size of acute myocardial infarction estimated from thallium scintiscans. *Circulation* 1977;56:72–78.

26. Maddahi J, Ganz W, Ninomiya K, et al. Myocardial salvage by intracoronary thrombolysis in evolving acute myocardial infarction. Evaluation using intracoronary injection of thallium-201. *Am Heart J* 1981;102:664.

27. Simoons ML, Wijns W, Balakumaran K, et al. The effect of intracoronary thrombolysis with streptokinase on myocardial thallium distribution and left ventricular function assessed by blood-pool scintigraphy. *Eur Heart J* 1982;3:433–440.

28. DeCoster PM, Melin JA, Detry J, et al. Coronary artery reperfusion in acute myocardial infarction: assessment by pre- and postintervention thallium-201 myocardial perfusion imaging. *Am J Cardiol* 1985;55:889.

29. Maddahi J, Weiss AT, Garcia EV, et al. Split-dose thallium-201 quantitative imaging for immediate post-reperfusion assessment of intravenous coronary thrombolysis. *Eur Heart J* 1985;6:127.

30. Beller GA. Role of myocardial perfusion imaging in evaluating thrombolytic therapy for acute myocardial infarction. *J Am Coll Cardiol* 1987;9:661.

31. Ritchie JL, Narahara KA, Trobaugh GB, et al. Thallium-201 myocardial imaging before and after coronary revascularization:

assessment of regional myocardial blood flow and graft patency. *Circulation* 1977;58:830–836.

32. Verani MS, Marcus ML, Spoto G, et al. Thallium-201 myocardial perfusion scintigrams in the evaluation of aorto-coronary saphenous bypass surgery. *J Nucl Med* 1977;19:765–772.

33. Hirzel HO, Nuesch K, Gruentzig AR, et al. Short- and long-term changes in myocardial perfusion after percutaneous transluminal coronary angioplasty assessed by thallium-201 exercise scintigraphy. *Circulation* 1981;63:1001–1007.

34. Verani MS, Tadros S, Raizner AE, et al. Quantitative analysis of thallium-201 uptake and washout before and after transluminal coronary angioplasty. *Int J Cardiol* 1986;13(2):109–124.

35. Hecht HS, Shaw RE, Bruce RT, et al. Usefulness of tomographic thallium-201 imaging for detection of restenosis after percutaneous transluminal angioplasty. *Am J Cardiol* 1990;66:1314–1318.

36. Hecht HS, Shaw RE, Chin HL, et al. Silent ischemia after coronary angioplasty: evaluation of restenosis and extent of ischemia in asymptomatic patients by tomographic thallium-201 exercise imaging and comparison with symptomatic patients. *J Am Coll Cardiol* 1991;17:670–677.

37. Plamas W, Bingham S, Diamond GA, et al. Incremental prognostic value of exercise thallium-201 myocardial single photon emission computed tomography late after coronary artery bypass. *J Am Coll Cardiol* 1995;25:403–409.

38. Wackers FJ, Lie KI, Liem KL, et al. Thallium scintigraphy in unstable angina pectoris. *Circulation* 1978;57:738–742.

39. Berger BC, Watson DD, Burwell LR, et al. Redistribution of thallium at rest in patients with stable and unstable angina and the effect of coronary artery bypass surgery. *Circulation* 1979;60:1114–1125.

40. Wackers FJ, Lie KI, Liem KL, et al. Potential value of thallium-201 scintigraphy as a means of selecting patients for the coronary care unit. *Br Heart J* 1979;41:111–117.

41. Brown K, Okada RD, Boucher CA, et al. Serial thallium-201 imaging at rest in patients with unstable and stable angina pectoris: relationship of myocardial perfusion at rest to presenting clinical syndrome. *Am Heart J* 1983;106:70–77.

42. Freeman MR, Williams AE, Chisholm RJ, et al. Role of resting thallium-201 perfusion in predicting coronary anatomy, left ventricular wall motion and hospital outcome in unstable angina pectoris. *Am Heart J* 1989;117:306–314.

43. van der Wieken LR, Kan G, Belfer AJ, et al. Thallium-201 scanning to decide CCU admission in patients with non-diagnostic electrocardiograms. *Int J Cardiol* 1983;4:285–299.
44. Hennemann PL, Mena IG, Rothstein RJ, et al. Evaluation of patients with chest pain and nondiagnostic ECG using thallium-201 myocardial planar imaging and technetium-99m first-pass radionuclide angiography in the emergency department. *Ann Emerg Med* 1992;21:545–550.
45. Mace SE. Thallium myocardial scanning in the emergency department evaluation of chest pain. *Am J Emerg Med* 1989;7:321–328.

Sestamibi and Other Technetium-99m Perfusion Agents

15

SUMMARY OF TECHNOLOGY

Clinical experience over the last two decades with patients with known or suspected CAD indicates that myocardial perfusion imaging can be used to identify patients with ACI occurring spontaneously or provoked by exercise or pharmacologic stress. Thallium-201 has been the only available tracer for this purpose until recently. Technetium-99m-labeled sestamibi (^{99m}Tc-sestamibi) has emerged during the past few years as an alternative myocardial perfusion agent with more advantageous imaging characteristics than thallium-201 (1–4). ^{99m}Tc-sestamibi, injected intravenously, is taken up by the myocardium in proportion to regional coronary blood flow. The regional distribution of the tracer can then be imaged with the use of a standard Anger camera (gamma camera). Unlike thallium-201, which washes out of the myocardium in proportion to blood flow, the initial myocardial distribution of ^{99m}Tc-sestamibi remains stable with time (1,4–6). Because sestamibi does not redistribute with time, images of initial blood flow at the time of injection can be acquired either shortly after administration or up to several hours later. This makes ^{99m}Tc-sestamibi a particularly useful and practical radiopharmaceutical for detecting myocardial ischemia in patients with spontaneous chest pain.

Perfusion abnormalities can often be detected by either thallium-201 or ^{99m}Tc-sestamibi for up to several hours after the last episode of chest pain in patients with cardiac ischemia (7,8). The reason for the persistent abnormality after cessation of symptoms may be the time that it takes cells to restore the impairment of cellular membrane function caused by transient myocardial ischemia (8,9).

Single-photon emission computed tomography (SPECT) imaging can be performed with ^{99m}Tc-sestamibi to better study myocardial perfusion and, with newer gated techniques, to look for segmental abnormalities of left ventricular wall-motion (hypokinesis, dyskinesis, or akinesis), failure of a portion of the left ventricle to thicken during systole, or frank systolic bulging of the affected myocardium (10). Ejection fraction can be measured accurately by gated tomographic sestamibi perfusion images (11). In experienced hands, ^{99m}Tc-sestamibi scintigraphy can provide valuable accurate diagnostic and prognostic information for patients presenting to the ED with symptoms consistent with ACI (3). If the resting ^{99m}Tc-sestamibi study is negative, a provocative stress study (exercise or pharmacologic) can be performed with ^{99m}Tc-sestamibi on adult patients with atypical symptoms, nondiagnostic ECGs, and no clinical or laboratory evidence (eg, serial ECGs and enzymes) of AMI to screen for the presence of hemodynamically significant CAD.

A number of new technetium-99m perfusion tracers have been developed that, like sestamibi, are not redistributed with time. These perfusion agents have potential value in the ED setting for evaluating patients with possible ACI. To date, data are available only for sestamibi, although the principles of sestamibi imaging in the ED may apply to the newer nonredistributed perfusion agents. This is the subject of ongoing investigation.

CRITIQUE
Scientific Basis

That the regional myocardial uptake of ^{99m}Tc-sestamibi is proportional to regional blood flow has been well established in a large number of laboratory conditions (5,6). In addition, the extraction and retention of sestamibi, a cationic compound, requires active processes at the level of the sarcolemma and mitochondrial membranes (12,13). Hence sestamibi uptake is a marker of cell membrane and mitochondrial integrity, and even if blood flow is restored, sestamibi is not retained in acutely or chronically infarcted myocardium (14).

The magnitude of sestamibi defects can be quantified, and sestamibi defect size has been shown to correlate with infarct size in human models of AMI (15,16). In addition, sestamibi defect size in human beings corresponds to other clinical estimates of infarct size, including CK release, regional wall-motion score, and final postinfarction left ventricular ejection fraction.

Clinical Practicality

Resting perfusion imaging with a portable gamma camera is practical in the ED setting. Whereas thallium-201 requires a cyclotron for production and is usually produced in a few central facilities and shipped to hospital nuclear medicine laboratories on a daily basis, ^{99m}Tc is produced onsite in most hospitals by means of elution from a generator and is available 24 hours a day. The major logistic problem with the use of ^{99m}Tc-sestamibi in this setting is the time required for preparation, which varies from 5 to 20 minutes.

Virtually all but the smallest hospitals in the United States have the ability to perform diagnostic quality myocardial perfusion imaging electively. In most cases, a nuclear medicine technician, nuclear medicine specialist, or a specially trained cardiologist or radiologist obtains the images. Diagnostic interpretation is usually provided by a nuclear medicine specialist or a specially trained cardiologist or radiologist. The problem with the routine use of ^{99m}Tc-sestamibi for the diagnosis of patients suspected of having an ACI syndrome in the ED is that the equipment is expensive, limiting its availability as standard equipment in an ED setting, and technologists and skilled physicians must be available 24 hours a day to obtain and read the images. The increasing use of teleradiology may help to overcome this problem.

Sestamibi can be made readily available in the ED setting. It is possible to keep two vials of sestamibi in the ED for use between 8 AM and midnight (one vial for the morning and one for the afternoon) by calibrating one vial for 30 mCi at noon and 1 for 30 mCi at 4 pm. This allows for 10 mCi of sestamibi to be available for injection until midnight, 7 days a week. ED personnel need to be educated in radiation-safety techniques, and care must be given to the injection of the agent during an episode of pain.

Nonetheless, patients must be transported to the nuclear medicine department for imaging. As noted, this can be 1 to 3 hours after the injection, so that the patient may be treated and stabilized before transport. Transport may not be practical in unstable patients.

Data from Prospective Clinical Trials in the ED Setting

No data are available from large prospective multicenter trials on the use of ^{99m}Tc-sestamibi in ACI/AMI. The subset of patients who would benefit from such imaging studies has not been defined. Nonetheless, some prospective evaluations have been done.

Studies of Test Sensitivity and Specificity: Hilton et al (17) studied 102 patients who were evaluated in the ED for angina-like chest pain who had normal or nondiagnostic ECGs. Sestamibi imaging was performed if it was ordered by the referring physician for clinical indications (not consecutive cases). Excluded were patients with historical or ECG evidence of prior infarction and those with atypical chest pain, ST-segment elevation, ST-segment depression of 1 mm or more, or new T-wave inversion. Multiple endpoints were considered: death, nonfatal infarction, and the need for immediate CABG, angioplasty, or thrombolysis. Seventy-nine patients were admitted to the hospital, and 23 (23%) were not. None of those who were not admitted had events or readmissions in the next 90 days.

According to the number of risk factors and their ECGs, patients were stratified into three risk categories that had event rates of 6% (in 33 low-risk patients), 11% (in 46 intermediate-risk patients), and 35% (in 23 high-risk patients). Combining intermediate- and high-risk groups, the presence of a patient in the higher risk category had a sensitivity of 88% and a specificity of 37% for predicting events. Events occurred in 15 patients (AMI in 12). Of 102 sestamibi scans, 70 (69%) were normal, and only 1 of these patients had an event (abnormal repeat scan, recurrent symptoms, CABG). Two of 15 patients with equivocal scans (13%) and 12 of 17 with abnormal scans (71%) had events. Combining the patients with equivocal and abnormal scans, there was a sensitivity of 94% and a specificity of 83% for predicting any event and a sensitivity and specificity of 100% and 83%, respectively, for predicting AMI.

Varetto et al (8) studied 274 consecutive CCU patients presenting to the ED with chest pain suspected to be of cardiac origin. In 208 patients, a diagnosis of noncardiac or cardiac pain was made in the ED. Sixty-six had presumed cardiac pain and a nondiagnostic ECG (normal, left bundle-branch block, or nonspecific ST-T-segment changes), were admitted to the CCU, and underwent sestamibi imaging (exclusions were those with definite noncardiac pain and cardiac pain with a diagnostic ECG). Because of a history of prior infarction (determined later), two patients were later excluded from analysis. Sestamibi imaging showed perfusion defects in 30 of 64 patients (47%); of these 30, AMI developed in 13 (43%),

14 (47%) had coronary disease on angiography but no infarct developed, and 3 (10%) were falsely positive (no coronary disease; one had left ventricular hemorrhage, one had aortic regurgitation, one was normal). There were no false negatives, as all 34 with negative sestamibi scans either had normal angiograms (22 [64%]) or negative exercise sestamibi scans (12 [36%]). Thus the sensitivity and specificity of resting sestamibi scanning were 100% and 92%, respectively. The negative and positive predictive values were 100% and 90%, respectively. However, if the two patients with prior infarction excluded ex post facto had been included, the specificity would have been lower. One important difference in this study is that the protocol did not require injection during pain (11 of 14 patients with coronary disease received sestamibi after cessation of pain). One limitation is that only patients admitted to the CCU were studied, which may represent an important selection bias; also, no one over age 70 was included.

Studies of the Clinical Impact of the Test's Actual Use: Three recent studies indicate that patients with possible ACI who have negative sestamibi studies in the ED setting have excellent outcomes. In the first study of 150 patients, reported by Hilton et al (18), there were no deaths, AMIs, or revascularization procedures over a 3-month period after the normal sestamibi scan. In the second study, by Weissman et al (19), the outcomes of 30 patients with chest pain with negative sestamibi studies in the ED, 26 of whom were discharged directly home from the ED, were excellent over an average 10-month follow-up time. There were no deaths, AMIs, or myocardial revascularization procedures in any of these patients. In contrast, among 20 patients with positive sestamibi studies in this series, 2 patients had AMIs and 3 patients underwent revascularization during the subsequent 10 months. In the third study, Tatum et al (20) reported 1,187 consecutive patients seen in the ED for a chief complaint of chest pain, with sestamibi imaging performed in the subset of patients with nondiagnostic ECG findings and probable or possible unstable angina. Sensitivity and specificity of the sestamibi scan for AMI were 100% and 78%, respectively. In patients with abnormal sestamibi scans, the risk for AMI was significantly higher than in those with normal scans (7% versus 0%, $P < 0.001$). During the next year, patients with abnormal sestamibi scans (n = 100) had an event rate of 42% (death, AMI, or revascularization), with 14% experiencing AMI and 9% cardiac death. In contrast, no patient with a normal sestamibi scan (n = 338) died or sustained an AMI during the 1-year follow-up period, and only 3% underwent myocardial revascularization.

Data from Other Clinical Studies

The limited data available for ^{99m}Tc-sestamibi for the early detection of ACI/AMI are encouraging. In one investigation of 45 patients hospitalized with a diagnosis of unstable angina, ^{99m}Tc-sestamibi imaging during an episode of chest pain had a 96% sensitivity and 79% specificity for significant CAD (21). The specificity was higher (84%) in patients who were studied after pain had been relieved. The negative predictive value of a normal ^{99m}Tc-sestamibi study was 94%.

It is also apparent from several studies that ^{99m}Tc-sestamibi has a number of quantitative uses for assessing the severity, as well as the presence, of AMI. Injection of sestamibi in AMI before giving thrombolytic agents may define the "area at risk," and repeat study after thrombolysis may quantitate myocardial salvage. In addition, the infarct-related artery can be predicted in patients with acute infarction and nondiagnostic ECGs.

Generalizability to Different Settings

One of the problems of ^{99m}Tc-sestamibi imaging is that its accuracy is highly dependent on the quality of the images obtained, the skill of the operator, and the knowledge and experience of the interpreter. It is unlikely that this technique will be widely applicable as a screening test in smaller community hospitals or rural ED settings.

Applicability to Population Subgroups, Including Women and Minorities

The principles of sestamibi imaging should apply well to both women and minorities. However, there are potential difficulties with interpretation of sestamibi images in some women because of photon attenuation artifacts caused by breast tissue, and in both sexes diaphragmatic attenuation may produce an inferior defect. Both of these attenuation artifacts may be recognized by experienced observers or by the use of newer gating techniques to assess wall motion and wall thickening (10). In general, because of the more favorable imaging characteristics of a ^{99m}Tc-based agent, sestamibi images have fewer interpretive errors as a result of such attenuation artifacts than do thallium-201 images.

There are no specific data on which to judge the accuracy or reliability of ^{99m}Tc-sestamibi imaging for detecting acute coronary ischemic syndromes in the ED setting in various population subgroups, including racial minorities, the elderly, and women.

Cost Considerations

The cost of the radiopharmaceutical is $100 to $150 per vial. Modern diagnostic-quality myocardial perfusion imaging equipment is relatively expensive, which limits its availability as a routine piece of equipment in the typical ED setting. Sestamibi imaging will increase the costs of the evaluation of the chest pain patient. Typical costs are in the range of $500 to $800 or more. Thus such imaging should be considered only in selected patient subgroups. As with any other test that might reduce unnecessary admissions, this cost would be offset by a significant reduction in admissions if the results of the above trials are borne out with further studies. Two preliminary studies suggest that sestamibi imaging in the ED in selected patient groups with chest pain would be cost-effective. Weissman et al (19) computed an average savings of $1,771 per patient in patients with nondiagnostic ECGs and allowed 66% of patients to be triaged to a less acute setting, 58% of whom were discharged home directly from the ED. Similarly, Radensky et al (22) computed a cost of $4,591 per patient using the sestamibi strategy compared with $5,514 per patient using no sestamibi. This was based on an 85% predictive accuracy in identifying patients with ACI using sestamibi compared with only 45% without sestamibi.

Special Concerns

Primarily, there is a need for prospective evaluation in clinical trials. There is a potential concern about the modest amount of radiation delivered to the patient. Also, see the disadvantages listed below.

Primary Advantages

Sestamibi imaging has become widely used in the past few years, and most nuclear medicine physicians and nuclear cardiologists have considerable training in its use and interpretation. The imaging equipment (a portable gamma camera) is available in most institutions. As noted previously, technetium is available in most hospital nuclear medicine laboratories at any time throughout the 24-hour day, unlike thallium-201.

In addition, ^{99m}Tc-sestamibi has ideal properties for gamma camera imaging. It has a shorter half-life compared with thallium-

201 (6 hours compared with 73 hours), which permits the administration of a higher dose (20 to 30 mCi). The higher dose, coupled with the higher energy of ^{99m}Tc, results in images with greater resolution than thallium-201 images. The lack of significant tracer redistribution after its initial myocardial uptake permits imaging either early after injection or at any time during the next 4 to 6 hours.

Doses of sestamibi can be made available in the ED to meet unpredictable needs. Kits can be delivered periodically (eg, monthly), and isotope would not have to be delivered every day or every other day as is the case with thallium-201.

Although the performance seen to date needs confirmation, sestamibi imaging's high sensitivity and specificity in the limited number of studies done to date is encouraging.

A potential logistic advantage is that the ED injection can be used for the resting study as the first part of an exercise sestamibi evaluation if the resting study is negative and the patient is stable, allowing for expeditious workup and early discharge of normal patients.

Primary Disadvantages

^{99m}Tc-sestamibi requires time for preparation and imaging, which could delay diagnosis and treatment. Also, imaging cannot be done for the first hour to allow for liver uptake to diminish. Further, usually patients must be moved from the ED to the nuclear medicine department for imaging (portable studies are not generally available).

Only experts specializing in nuclear medicine are qualified to evaluate the scans (although the increasing use of teleradiology may help overcome the problem with the lack of these personnel in smaller institutions). Also, ED personnel must be trained in radiation-safety techniques to provide safe storage and injection of the material.

The true sensitivity and specificity are still unknown (not enough studies).

Sestamibi imaging is expensive and costs more than thallium-201.

SUMMARY AND RECOMMENDATIONS

The use of resting radionuclide imaging for the diagnosis of ACI/AMI in the ED should be restricted to specific and limited

Table 15-1   Sestamibi and Other Technetium-99m Perfusion Agents

ED Diagnostic Performance		ED Clinical Impact	
Quality of Evidence	Accuracy	Quality of Evidence	Impact
C	+++	NK	NK

conditions in which the clinical triad of history, ECG changes, and enzymatic/laboratory measurements is not available or is unreliable. Such imaging may be helpful, for example, in patients with equivocal chest pain histories and nondiagnostic ECG findings. The applicability of this imaging modality depends primarily on logistic issues. ^{99m}Tc-sestamibi is an excellent perfusion tracer, with advantageous physical characteristics compared with thallium-201. Its availability, excellent imaging properties, and stable tracer distribution with time make it a practical agent for ED use. Additional technetium-99m–based perfusion agents are available or soon will be available that share many of sestamibi's properties and may also be suitable for imaging in patients with suspected ACI. Although large-scale trials are lacking, the available data (in relatively small numbers of patients) indicate that ^{99m}Tc-sestamibi is a promising agent for use in the ED evaluation of selected patients with chest pain. Its use to date has been limited to a handful of centers that have studied patients who were judged to be at relatively high risk of having ACI, particularly those having chest pain at the time of the study. It is unclear whether the technique will be of value as a screening test in lower risk ED patients without ongoing chest pain or when used by less-experienced interpreters. However, until more evidence is available, it cannot yet be recommended at this stage for general use.

The results of the Working Group's final ratings of the quality of evidence evaluating this technology and of its ED diagnostic performance and clinical impact are shown in Table 15-1.

REFERENCES

1. Zaret BL, Wackers FJ. Nuclear cardiology. *N Engl J Med* 1993;329:775–783, 855–863.
2. Van Train KF, Garcia EV, Maddahi J, et al. Multicenter trial validation for quantitative analysis of same-day rest-stress technetium-99m-sestamibi myocardial tomograms. *J Nucl Med* 1994;35:609–618.

3. Berman DS, Kiat HS, Van Train KF, et al. Myocardial perfusion imaging with technetium-99m-sestamibi: comparative analysis of available imaging protocols. *J Nucl Med* 1994;35:681–688.
4. Ritchie JL, Bateman TM, Bonow RO, et al. Guidelines for clinical use of cardiac radionuclide imaging. A report of the American Heart Association/American College of Cardiology Task Force on Assessment of Diagnostic and Therapeutic Cardiovascular Procedures. *Circulation* 1995;91:1278–1302.
5. Okada RD, Glover D, Gaffney T, et al. Myocardial kinetics of technetium-99m hexakis-2-methoxy-2-methylpropyl-isonitrile. *Circulation* 1988;77:491–498.
6. Glover D, Okada RD. Myocardial kinetics of Tc-MIBI in canine myocardium after dipyridamole. *Circulation* 1990;81:628–636.
7. Wackers FJ, Lie KI, Liem KL, et al. Potential value of thallium-201 scintigraphy as a means of selecting patients for the coronary care unit. *Br Heart J* 1979;41:111–117.
8. Varetto T, Cantalupi D, Altieri A, et al. Emergency room technetium-99m sestamibi imaging to rule out acute myocardial ischemic events in patients with nondiagnostic electrocardiograms. *J Am Coll Cardiol* 1993;22:1804–1808.
9. Gregoire J, Theroux P. Detection and assessment of unstable angina using myocardial perfusion imaging: comparison between technetium-99m sestamibi SPECT and 12-lead electrocardiogram. *Am J Cardiol* 1990;66:42–46.
10. Chua T, Kiat H, Germano G, et al. Gated technetium-99m-sestamibi for simultaneous assessment of stress myocardial perfusion, postexercise regional function and myocardial viability: correlation with echocardiography and rest thallium scintigraphy. *J Am Coll Cardiol* 1994;23:1107–1114.
11. Germano G, Kiat HS, Kavanaagh PB, et al. Automatic quantification of ejection fraction from gated myocardial perfusion SPECT. *J Nucl Med* 1995;36:2138–2147.
12. Beanlands RSB, Dawood F, Wen WH, et al. Are the kinetics of technetium-99m methoxyisobutyl isonitrile affected by cell metabolism and viability? *Circulation* 1990;82:1802–1814.
13. Piwnica-Worms D, Kronauge JF, Chiu ML. Uptake and retention of hexakis (2-methoxyisobutyl isonitrile) technetium in cultured myocardial cells: mitochondrial and plasma membrane potential dependence. *Circulation* 1990;82:1826–1838.
14. Bonow RO, Dilsizian V. Thallium-201 and technetium 99m ses-

tamibi for assessing viable myocardium. *J Nucl Med* 1992;33: 815–818.

15. Gibbons RJ, Verani MS, Behrenbeck T, et al. Feasibility of tomographic 99m-Tc-hexakis-2-methoxy-2-methylpropyl-isonitrile for the assessment of myocardial area at risk and the effect of treatment in acute myocardial infarction. *Circulation* 1989;80:1277–1286.

16. Christian TF, Schwartz RS, Gibbons RJ. Determinants of infarct size in reperfusion therapy for acute myocardial infarction. *Circulation* 1992;86:81–90.

17. Hilton TC, Thompson RC, Williams HJ, et al. Technetium-99m sestamibi myocardial perfusion imaging in the emergency room evaluation of chest pain. *J Am Coll Cardiol* 1994;23:1016–1022.

18. Hilton TC, Stowers SA, Fulmer H. Ninety day follow-up of emergency department patients with chest pain and normal or non-diagnostic ECG who undergo acute cardiac imaging with Tc-99m-sestamibi (abstract). *J Am Coll Cardiol* 1995;25:192A.

19. Weissman IA, Dickinson C, Dworkin H, et al. Emergency center myocardial perfusion SPECT—long-term follow-up: cost-effective imaging providing diagnostic and prognostic information (abstract). *J Nucl Med* 1995;36:P88.

20. Tatum JL, Jesse RL, Kontos MC, et al. A comprehensive strategy for the evaluation and triage of the chest pain patient. *Ann Emerg Med* (in press).

21. Bilodeau L, Theroux P, Gregoire J, et al. Technetium-99m sestamibi topography in patients with spontaneous chest pain: correlations with clinical, electrocardiographic and angiographic findings. *J Am Coll Cardiol* 1991;1:1684–1691.

22. Radensky PW, Stowers S, Hilton TC, et al. Cost-effectiveness of acute myocardial perfusion imaging with TC99m sestamibi for risk stratification of emergency room patients with acute chest pain (abstract). *Circulation* 1994;90:I–528.

Conclusions and Recommendations

16

The previous sections summarize the Working Group's reviews of current diagnostic technologies for ACI and AMI in the ED. To make recommendations for clinical practice, the Working Group's charge included specifying the extent to which there are data that demonstrate each technology's effectiveness in actual use in the ED setting. These assessments of the quality and magnitude of reported results and the resultant recommendations are summarized in this concluding section.

As detailed in the first section of this report, as a first step in the Working Group's evaluations, each technology's primary diagnostic purpose in the ED was identified, for which its literature and reported performance would be judged. Three primary purposes were identified, and the technologies were categorized as follows: 1) *The detection of ACI in the general ED population in order to accurately discriminate patients with ACI from those without ACI among those presenting with symptoms consistent with ACI:* standard ECG, the original ACI predictive instrument, the Goldman chest pain protocol, the ACI-TIPI, and other predictive instruments. 2) *The early identification of ACI, particularly in those with ST-segment elevation due to AMI:* prehospital ECG. 3) *The detection of ACI in certain subgroups:* continuous ECG, nonstandard ECG leads, body-surface mapping, CK and other biochemical tests for AMI, echocardiography, thallium scanning, sestamibi and other technetium-99m perfusion agents, and ECG exercise stress testing.

As also detailed earlier, a formal process of review and evaluation of the scientific literature related to these technologies was based on literature searches supplemented by the panelists' knowledge of the literature and ongoing research. (In each technology's section, published abstracts that have not yet appeared as peer-reviewed articles are reviewed and are mentioned in the recommendations below, but to avoid selection bias, such preliminary results are not included in the final ratings in the summary table of the literature [Table 16-1].) In reviewing available data, results were considered only if they came from work done *in the emergency setting*; results coming from other settings (eg, the CCU) were used only if no ED-based data were available, and then only as suggestive rather than definitive data.

On the basis of these reviews, each technology, for its primary purpose, was rated in terms of its *diagnostic performance* for identifying ACI/AMI in actual use and its demonstrated *clinical impact* on ED care when used in practice. Performance in each of these two dimensions was rated as: +++, very accurate/large clinical impact; ++, moderately accurate/medium impact; +, modestly accurate/small impact; NK, not known; or NE, not effective. Also, the quality of evidence provided by the relevant studies relating to these measures was rated as A, prospective controlled clinical trials of high quality (eg, large multicenter trials with concurrent controls); B, substantial clinical studies; C, limited studies or evidence (eg, case series, small clinical studies); or NK, not known (eg, expert opinion or case reports only). These ratings, as assigned to the reviewed technologies, are summarized at the end of this section in Table 16-1.

Clinical Recommendations

Ideally, recommendations for the use of the reviewed technology would be based on demonstrated impact on care, but such evidence is currently available, or even pending, for only a small minority (1,2). There is a clear need for more data on these technologies' actual ED diagnostic performance and especially on their clinical impact on emergency care. Understanding multiple types of tests and their contribution to the diagnosis of ACI when they are performed in series or parallel is a complex undertaking. Because this has not been studied, clinical judgment is often required to reach diagnostic conclusions. However, to provide some clinical recommendations for current practice, the Working Group attempted to arrive at conclusions based on currently available data for each technology. To make clear which recommendations were based on which levels of evidence, these clinical recommendations are listed below by category of their level of supportive data.

Table 16-1 Summary Ratings of Diagnostic Technologies for ACI for ED Use

Technology	Primary Diagnostic Use	ED Diagnostic Performance		ED Clinical Impact	
		Quality of Evidence	Accuracy	Quality of Evidence	Impact
Standard ECG	G	A	++	Standard of care	Standard of care
Original ACI predictive instrument	G	A	+++	A	+++
ACI-TIPI	G	A	+++	C*	+*
Prehospital ECG	E	A	++	B	+
Goldman chest pain protocol	G	A	For AMI: +++ For UAP: NE	B	NK/NE
CK, multiple tests over time	S	A	For AMI: +++ For UAP: NE	NK	NK
Sestamibi	S	C	+++	NK	NK
CK, single test	S	A	For AMI: + For UAP: NE	NK	NK

ECG exercise stress test	S	C	+	C	NK/NE
Echocardiogram	S	B	+	NK	NK
Other computer-based decision aids	G	B	+	NK	NK
Troponin–T and troponin–I	S	B	For AMI: ++ For UAP: NE	NK	NK
Myoglobin	S	B	For AMI: + For UAP: NE	NK	NK
Nonstandard ECG leads	S	C	+	NK	NK
Thallium scanning	S	C	NK/NE	NK	NK/NE
Body-surface mapping	S	NK	NK	NK	NK
Continuous 12-lead ECG	S	NK	NK	NK	NK

AMI = acute myocardial infarction; UAP = unstable angina pectoris; G = general detection of ACI; E = early detection; S = detection in subgroup.
Diagnostic rating: A = high-quality clinical studies; B = substantial clinical studies; C = limited studies; NK = not known; NE = not effective.
Clinical impact rating: +++ = very accurate/large clinical impact; ++ = moderately accurate/medium impact; + = modestly accurate/small impact; NK = not known; NE = not effective; ★ abstract and pending reports are not included in the ratings.
Technologies are listed in order of the Working Group's ratings of diagnostic accuracy and demonstrated clinical impact and alphabetically among equivalent ratings, with the exception of standard ECG, which is considered to be a standard of care.

Summary of Clinical Recommendations Based on Diagnostic Performance and Clinical Impact:

Recommendations regarding the use of a technology should be based on both ED diagnostic performance and clinical impact data obtained in high-quality or substantial studies. Of the various diagnostic technologies evaluated in the 14 sections, however, only 5 met this highly desirable standard of evaluation.

The original ACI predictive instrument was found to be excellent for diagnostic performance (+ + +) and substantial clinical impact (+ + +) in a high-quality prospective multicenter trial (A) for both forms of ACI (unstable angina and AMI). Its accuracy and demonstrated improvement in ED triage make it possible to recommend it for general use in the ED evaluation and triage of patients with symptoms suggestive of ACI. Its main drawback has been that its use requires a programmed calculator or chart, which has been an obstacle to its widespread use. This may be overcome by its successor, the ACI-TIPI, which is incorporated into and reported as part of the header printout on a standard 12-lead ECG.

The second diagnostic technology on which there are studies of both diagnostic performance and clinical impact is the *ACI-TIPI*, although the largest clinical trial of impact is available only in abstract form. It has diagnostic performance (+ + +) comparable to that of the original ACI predictive instrument, on the basis of multicenter prospective studies (A), and the ECG-based ACI-TIPI has ease of use. On the basis of published clinical trials but not including the results of a large prospective trial published to date only in abstract form, its quality of evidence is a C, and clinical impact rating is a +. More definitive recommendations regarding its general use await the full publication of the results of the multicenter trial.

The prehospital ECG was found to have good (+ +) diagnostic performance on the basis of evidence from high-quality prospective studies (A). However, this technology was judged to have a small clinical impact (+) on the basis of substantial clinical studies (A). It was the impression of the Working Group, on the basis of these results, that although this technology has promise, it will probably be realized in areas with long EMS transport times. Thus, until more evidence is obtained, its general use cannot be recommended.

The fourth technology for which data are available on both its ED diagnostic performance and clinical impact is the *Goldman chest pain protocol*. An important caveat, however, is that this protocol was designed only for AMI detection and not the more general detection of ACI in the form of unstable angina. Its diagnostic performance for AMI has been demonstrated to be excellent (+ + +) in multicenter high-quality studies (A). However, in a high-quality prospective study (B), it has not had a demonstrable impact on clinical care (NK-NE), and thus at this point its general use cannot be recommended.

The final diagnostic technology, the *ECG exercise stress test*, a different extension of the standard ECG, has also been evaluated to some extent in the ED. Its diagnostic performance for CAD in this setting has been only modest. Given this, and that its actual impact on triage has received only limited testing, its routine ED use cannot be recommended.

Clinical Recommendations Based on Demonstrated Diagnostic Performance but Without Data on Clinical Impact: For all but five of the technologies reviewed above there was some published evidence of diagnostic performance but no studies of actual clinical impact (ie, all evidence grades were NK for clinical impact). The Working Group strongly advises that, with the exception of the standard 12-lead ECG (see immediately below), diagnostic performance alone is an insufficient basis for recommendation for general use. This is from the long experience of numerous examples of technologies that have excellent or good diagnostic performance but negligible or even negative clinical impact when tested under conditions of actual use (1–4).

The *standard 12-lead ECG* has been shown in many studies to have very good, although not perfect, diagnostic performance in the ED. However, despite its key role in the diagnosis of ACI in the ED, it has not been demonstrated to have impact on care in the ED setting other than its central role in other technologies such as the ACI predictive instruments described above. In fact, given that the ECG is part of standard ED evaluation, in the view of the Working Group, a trial to demonstrate its impact would be neither necessary nor ethical. Indeed, the 12-lead ECG should be part of the very initial evaluation of any ED or EMS patient with symptoms suggestive of ACI.

Although they have not as of yet been demonstrated to actually improve clinical care in the ED, *blood biochemical tests of myocardial necrosis, particularly CK*, including a variety of assay types and protocols, have undergone prospective testing of their diagnostic performance for the detection of AMI. Available data suggest that the use of a *single CK-MB* test yields performance insufficient for use in ED triage but that the use of *multiple CK-MB* tests over several or more hours has very good diagnostic performance for AMI. Although less complete, the data for *troponin* also suggest that performance of a single test is not satisfactory. The use of multiple tests over time may improve diagnostic performance. The one other biochemical test that has undergone considerable testing is *myoglobin*, but its performance has not yet defined its exact role as an early marker of AMI. Finally, neither myoglobin nor CK detect UAP, which raises the possibility of missing this form of ACI if triage is dependent on such tests. This is one of the reasons that in the absence of prospective trials of the impact of this technology on ED triage (level of admission or discharge), these tests cannot yet be recommended for general ED triage use at this time, although they are very useful for in-hospital care.

Echocardiography, well studied in other settings, has undergone several studies in the ED, which have generally shown modest diagnostic performance for initial ED evaluation. Given this, and that its actual impact on ED care has not been evaluated, this technology cannot be recommended for general ED use at this time.

Radionuclide imaging, although generally used in non–ED settings, has undergone some study of diagnostic performance in the ED. *Thallium scanning* is less appropriate for ED use than sestamibi, has not been evaluated in ED use and cannot be recommended. *Sestamibi and other technetium-99m perfusion agents* have been studied in the ED setting, and although the overall diagnostic performance of sestamibi has been promising, it has not been sufficiently tested to recommend its general ED use. Whether sestamibi will be found to be more helpful when evaluated for special subgroups, and when tested for its actual impact on care, remains to be seen. At this point, its general ED use cannot be recommended.

As an extension of the standard ECG, *nonstandard ECG leads* have undergone some limited testing in the ED for detecting ACI, and another prospective trial was just completed. The quality (C) of published data at this point does not provide sufficient evidence of diagnostic utility. This may be altered by the just-finished trial. In addition, its impact on care has not been tested, and thus nonstandard ECG leads cannot yet be recommended for general use.

Although reported in several case studies in EDs or suggested in a preliminary way in discussions of work done in other settings such as the CCU, *continuous ECG* and *body-surface mapping* have not been tested with regard to their diagnostic performance in general ED use or for their impact on ED care, and these cannot be recommended for general use at this time.

RECOMMENDATIONS FOR RESEARCH

Although the primary purpose of this report is to provide clinical recommendations, Table 16-1 makes it clear that there is currently a great lack of research results related to the diagnostic performance and especially the clinical impact of these most important technologies for the emergency evaluation of the most common cause of death in our country. Further diagnostic trials addressing both their accuracy and impact are critical to the NHAAP mission to improve rapidity and effectiveness of care for emergency cardiac patients. Additionally, the evaluation of diagnostic approaches integrating multiple technologies (such as panels of different biochemical markers) or of multiple modalities (such as combining ECG, imaging, and biochemical tests) is needed. In doing this, it will be important to understand the incremental contribution of each modality. In this context, further investigation is needed of the potential utility of computer-based decision aids and analytic programs for integrating and presenting different forms of information.

With more than 6 million patients yearly in this country presenting to the ED with chest pain or analogous symptoms (5,6) and with the care of those unnecessarily admitted to cardiac care costing on the order of $3 billion a year (7) while approximately 20,000 ED patients are inappropriately sent home each year (8,9), there is little question that such studies of ways to improve diagnostic and triage performance would be an excellent investment financially and would substantially improve medical care. The Working Group strongly recommends that such studies be supported far more than has been the case to date.

REFERENCES

1. Selker HP. Coronary care unit triage decision aids: how do we know when they work? *Am J Med* 1989;87:491–493.
2. McCarthy BD, Wong JB, Selker HP. Detecting acute cardiac ischemia in the emergency department: a review of the literature. *J Gen Intern Med* 1990;5:365–373.
3. American College of Emergency Physicians (ACEP). Policy

Statement—Prehospital Use of Thrombolytic Agents. Approved by the ACEP Board of Directors, October 1993.

4. Lee TH, Pearson SD, Johnson PA, et al. Failure of information as an intervention to modify clinical management: a time-series trial in patients with acute chest pain. *Ann Intern Med* 1995; 122:434–437.

5. The SUPPORT Principal Investigators. A controlled trial to improve care for seriously ill hospitalized patients: the Study to Understand Prognosis and Preferences for Outcomes and Risks of Treatment (SUPPORT). *JAMA* 1995;274(20):1591–1598.

6. McCaig L. National Hospital Ambulatory Medical Care Survey. 1992 emergency department summary. *Advance Data* 1994;245:1–12.

7. Pozen MW, D'Agostino RB, Selker HP, et al. A predictive instrument to improve coronary-care-unit admission practices in acute ischemic heart disease: a prospective multicenter trial. *N Engl J Med* 1984;310:1273–1278.

8. Fineberg HV, Scadden D, Goldman L. Care of patients with a low probability of acute myocardial infarction: cost-effectiveness of alternatives to coronary care unit admission. *N Engl J Med* 1984;310:1301–1307.

9. McCarthy BD, Beshansky JR, D'Agostino RB, et al. Missed diagnoses of acute myocardial infarction in the emergency department: results from a multicenter study. *Ann Emerg Med* 1993;22:579–582.

10. Lee TH, Rouan GW, Weisberg MC, et al. Clinical characteristics and natural history of patients with acute myocardial infarction sent home from the emergency room. *Am J Cardiol* 1987;60(4):219–224.

Index

Acute cardiac ischemia (ACI)
  predictive instrument,
  65–76
  advantages of, 74–75
  clinical impact of, 71–73
  clinical practicality of, 70
  cost of, 74
  data from other clinical studies of,
    73
  disadvantages of, 75
  generalizability to different settings
    of, 73–74
  incorporation into ECG of, 66–
    67
  for population subgroups, 74
  probabilities on, 68–69
  quality of evidence on, 75
  recommendations for, 75–76, 174,
    176
  scientific basis of, 70
  sensitivity and specificity of, 71,
    72
  special concerns with, 74
  technology of, 65–66
Acute cardiac ischemia time-insensitive predictive instrument
  (ACI-TIPI), 77–90
  advantages of, 89
  clinical impact of, 84–86
  clinical practicality of, 81
  cost of, 88

data from other clinical studies of,
    87
  disadvantages of, 89
  generalizability to different settings
    of, 87
  for population subgroups, 88
  quality of evidence on, 90
  recommendations for, 89–90, 174,
    176
  scientific basis of, 79, 81
  sensitivity and specificity of,
    81–83
  special concerns with, 88–89
  technology of, 77–79
Admissions practice, ACI predictive
  instrument and, 72–73

Belgian Eminase Prehospital Study
  (BEPS), 21–22
Biochemical tests, 125–135. *See also*
  Creatine kinase (CK)
  advantages of, 133
  clinical impact of, 130
  clinical practicality of, 128
  cost of, 131
  data from other clinical studies of,
    130
  disadvantages of, 134
  generalizability to different settings
    of, 131
  quality of evidence on, 135